The
LEAN
BELLY
Prescription

The
LEAN
BELLY
Prescription

The Fast And Foolproof Diet and Weight-Loss Plan From America's Top Urgent-Care Doctor

TRAVIS STORK, M.D.,
HOST OF TV'S *THE DOCTORS*,
WITH PETER MOORE,
EDITOR OF *MEN'S HEALTH*®

RODALE

NOTICE

This book is intended as a reference volume only, not as a medical manual. The information given here is designed to help you make informed decisions about your health. It is not intended as a substitute for any treatment that may have been prescribed by your doctor. If you suspect that you have a medical problem, we urge you to seek competent medical help.

The information in this book is meant to supplement, not replace, proper exercise training. All forms of exercise pose some inherent risks. The editors and publisher advise readers to take full responsibility for their safety and know their limits. Before practicing the exercises in this book, be sure that your equipment is well-maintained, and do not take risks beyond your level of experience, aptitude, training, and fitness. The exercise and dietary programs in this book are not intended as a substitute for any exercise routine or dietary regimen that may have been prescribed by your doctor. As with all exercise and dietary programs, you should get your doctor's approval before beginning.

Mention of specific companies, organizations, or authorities in this book does not imply endorsement by the author or publisher, nor does mention of specific companies, organizations, or authorities imply that they endorse this book, its author, or the publisher.

Internet addresses and telephone numbers given in this book were accurate at the time it went to press.

Rodale books may be purchased for business or promotional use or for special sales. For information, please write to:
Special Markets Department, Rodale Inc., 733 Third Avenue, New York, NY 10017

Men's Health is a registered trademark of Rodale Inc.

Printed in the United States of America
Rodale Inc. makes every effort to use acid-free ⊗, recycled paper ♲.

Book design by Mike Smith,
with George Karabotsos, design director of *Men's Health* Books
Photographs by Tom MacDonald

Library of Congress Cataloging-in-Publication Data
Stork, Travis.
    The lean belly prescription : the fast and foolproof diet and weight-loss plan from America's top urgent-care doctor / Travis Stork with Peter Moore, editor of Men's Health.
        p. cm.
    ISBN 978-1-60961-023-4 (hardcover)
    1. Weight loss. 2. Abdomen. I. Moore, Peter. II. Title.
    RM222.2.S76 2011
    613.2'5--dc22   2010040008
Distributed to the trade by Macmillan
                        4 6 8 10 9 7 5 3   hardcover

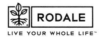

RODALE
LIVE YOUR WHOLE LIFE™

We inspire and enable people to improve their lives and the world around them.

To the lean you,
the real you—a person who's free from
all that weighs you down and
holds you back and threatens your health.
Together, we can lift your burden.

CONTENTS

The Last Word in Weight Loss

I am not a doctor. Nor do I play one on TV.

But Travis Stork, M.D., is—in real life *and* on TV. As an emergency-medicine physician in Nashville, he mans the E.R., caring for the injured and the ill, making split-second decisions that often spell the difference between life and death. As one of the hosts of TV's *The Doctors*, he spreads the gospel of good health to millions of Americans from a TV studio in Los Angeles. Wherever Travis Stork goes, he changes lives for the better.

With this book, he wants to change yours, too—in just 4 weeks! So if you're looking to get a lean, flat belly—and the improved health, longevity, and self-confidence that come with it—you've come to the right place.

Dr. Travis's *Lean Belly Prescription* might be the easiest, most sensible weight-loss-and-lifestyle book I've ever read. And I've read them all. As editor-in-chief of *Men's Health*, editorial direc-tor of *Women's Health*, and the author of the *Eat This, Not That!* series of books, I spend my days, and more often than I'd like, my nights—listening to experts, poring over studies, and testing the latest and greatest health, fitness, and weight-loss theories. But I've never come across a program as effective and as easy to stick to as this one. When it comes to slimming down, toning up, and (at last!) having the firm, lean belly you've always wanted, this book might just be the final word.

See, the problem with most weight-loss plans is that they're not flexible, they're not realistic, and they're not adaptable to the way real people live their real lives. But *The Lean Belly Prescription* is different. Dr. Travis might call his belly-fat cure a "prescription," but it's actually the most flexible program you'll ever find. His revolutionary PICK 3 TO LEAN plan doesn't require you to give up your favorite foods or to stop doing anything you love to do. Instead, he gives you a broad range of dietary changes you can make, based on your favorite foods and how you like to eat them. In a sense, you design your own weight-loss strategy. And if you get tired of following it? Heck, you just go back and design a different one!

But it's not just the genius of the plan that's so terrific. What's most touching and telling about this book is Dr. Travis's motivation for writing it. Simply put, he got tired of patching up patients in the E.R. only to send them back out into a world where two-thirds of them will live their lives as overweight or obese people. Dr. Travis wants to change lives, not just for an hour on the television, or one night in the emergency room. With *The Lean Belly Prescription*, Dr. Travis has a much bigger mission: He wants to change people's lives forever.

Starting with yours!

David Zinczenko

Editor-in-chief of *Men's Health*
and editorial director of *Women's Health*

ACKNOWLEDGMENTS

I would like to acknowledge my family and friends. Without your support I would not be on this mission to promote health beyond the E.R. You have taught me that friendliness, hard work, and honesty can never be taken away.

To the entire team at *The Doctors*, who work tirelessly to prove that an hour of television can and does make a POSITIVE difference. Thank you!

To all of my peers and mentors in medicine, many of whom don't get the credit they so greatly deserve.

I'd like to specifically acknowledge the efforts and creativity of Peter Moore, David Zinczenko, and the entire team at Rodale and *Men's Health* for giving this book direction, meaning, and most importantly, information that will not only save lives, but also improve them. Thanks go to the Rodale books team, led by Karen Rinaldi, and Chris Krogermeier and Sara Cox; the *Men's Health* and *Women's Health* books juggernaut, including Stephen Perrine, George Karabotsos, Debbie McHugh, Erin Williams, and designer Mike Smith; Laura Roberson, for her wide-ranging research; Paul Kita, Maria Masters, and David Schipper; fitness models Jackson Bloore and Megan Hoffman, stylist Kathy Kalafut, and hair/makeup stylist Colleen Kobrick-Kuehne; copy editors Nancy Elgin, Susan Hindman, Dave Caruso, and Claire McCrea; and Adam Campbell, author of *The Big Book of Exercises*, and Jeff Csatari, author of the *Belly Off! Diet*, for their many contributions. A personal thank you goes to Lisa Furnish, Mel Berger, and Scott Zolke.

And lastly, I would like to acknowledge anyone reading this book. May this be your first step on a lifelong journey toward health and happiness.

Peter Moore adds:

I'd like to thank my mom, Dorothy Moore; my late father, Richard Moore; my wife, Claire; and my sons Jake and Tyler, with whom I've proved and re-proved the studies that show how family activity builds the most important muscle: the heart.

The Killer Fat Within

*America's top urgent-care doctor targets
"killer fat"—the greatest risk to your health,
your life, and even your bank account—
with a revolutionary new 4-week prescription that
will grant you a lean belly for life!*

IT'S ANOTHER SATURDAY NIGHT IN THE E.R.

I haven't been too busy—an unexplained rash here, a wrist sprain there—which can mean only one thing: It's just a matter of time before somebody out there gets seriously hurt.

And sure enough, the PA system barks a warning, announcing an auto accident with multiple injuries. I leap to my feet and abandon a cup of coffee that I won't return to for several hours. Who needs caffeine when you're pumping high-test adrenaline? I've been preparing for moments like this for my whole medical career: getting my E.R. patients through the "golden hour," the critical 60 minutes that determine whether they will live or die.

I hear the sirens wailing as the ambulances near Vanderbilt University Medical Center in Nashville, Tennessee, where I'm on call in the E.R. whenever I'm not in Los Angeles hosting *The Doctors*. If you think hosting a TV show watched by millions of people must be stressful, then you haven't spent a night in the E.R.

Two ambulances arrive at the door, and in a flash the victims roll down the hallways and into my care. In the E.R., I have to determine immediately what's wrong and figure out how I can help the next patient who arrives, often on death's doorstep.

So what is one of the first vital signs I check? How much they weigh.

C'mon, Dr. Travis, you're thinking. *You don't check for a pulse or blood pressure? You don't check for missing limbs or scan the report compiled by the ambulance personnel?* Well, sure, I'm looking at a lot of things simultaneously, but often one of the most important indicators of how well a patient will manage a health crisis is how much excess weight he or she is carrying. In fact, research suggests that obese people are 37 percent more likely to die from injuries sustained in a car crash than people of ideal weight.

The patient who just arrived in Trauma Bay 1 is an unfortunate example of that. He's more than 50 pounds overweight, and evidence retrieved from the car indicates that he was eating behind the wheel when the accident happened. His body is under siege—not just by the injuries he sustained in his accident, but by the myriad complications brought on by all that belly fat. In fact, visceral fat—the most dangerous kind of fat, the fat inside your abdomen that packs internal organs in a toxic soup of goop—literally attacks the people who are lugging it around all day. It's one of the primary causes of the diseases that haunt our lives: Heart disease. Stroke. Diabetes. Cancer. Arthritis. And that's if you stay out of car accidents and other mishaps. If you're injured, the added weight actually fights your body's natural healing powers.

In the short time I have with people in medical emergencies, my focus is obviously the acute injury or illness. I may help a patient survive his most recent accident, but the ultimate accident that costs many of my patients their lives isn't really any accident at all. It's a lifetime of making unhealthy choices, often scores of them each day, that leads to a premature death.

And that's why I wrote this book. Like many of my fellow doctors, I find it difficult to discharge my patients back into a world where they'll grow more obese, more out of shape, more frustrated by their struggles with their weight. It's heartbreaking to see them back in the E.R. 2 years later, with another heart attack, another stroke, another obesity-related complication. I have the power to write them a prescription for medicine, but what I really want is to write them a prescription for a better life.

And now I have.

WHY WE NEED A LEAN BELLY PRESCRIPTION

In the crazed, adrenaline-fueled moments I have with E.R. patients, I try to give them the best lifestyle advice I can: why they need to watch what they eat, why exercise is so important, why making small changes to their daily activities will have a profound impact on their health—how they look, how they feel, how they live. And often, I'm met with a blank stare, a shrug, and a noncommittal murmur. "Lifestyle changes" seem hard, especially when a doctor is trying to explain them to you in 5 minutes or less. In fact, more often than not, my patients will look at me and ask one question:

"Doc, can't you just give me a prescription?"

Well, yes. I can. Not for a weight-loss pill you can pop, and not for an elective surgery that will trim you down suddenly. (Both have terrible potential side effects and spotty long-term track records.) Instead, I've written a prescription that simply, effectively, and nearly effortlessly strips away pounds, focusing on your biggest enemy and mine—belly fat.

I've created a list of eight life-altering dietary changes that will burn away belly fat with shocking speed. I call them "The Laws of Leanness." But you don't actually have to make all eight changes. In fact, you don't even have to make half of them. These lifestyle tweaks are so powerful, so dramatically effective, that if you make just three of them—your three favorite, whichever ones you want—you can drop up to 15 pounds in 4 weeks or less. I call it PICK 3 TO LEAN. And the best part? You'll keep losing after those first 4 weeks—15, even 20 pounds, you decide—and you'll *never* gain it back!

And I've based these dietary secrets not on foods I want you to give up, but on foods I want you to enjoy. For example:

• Love pasta and rice? I'll show you how to eat them and still lose 24 percent more belly fat than traditional "dieters" do.

• Crazy about milk shakes? Then drink two a day (with my special recipe) and strip away pounds.

• Enjoy snacking? I'll show you how to build several snacks every single day that will fuel weight loss while keeping you satisfied.

Combined with your choice of easy, effective activity programs, which you'll also find outlined in this book—you won't think of these as "exercise"—your PICK 3 choices will begin to strip away belly fat almost from day one.

How do I know that? Because I've based this prescription on the latest science, on results that have been proven by the top researchers in America and abroad. And I've based it on my experience as a medical doctor, watching what works, and what doesn't, in the real world. I've seen these strategies succeed for my patients, sure, but I've also seen them work for friends and family members who have turned to me for help. Now I want to include you in that group of happy, grateful, newly skinny people.

BLAST FAT, STAT!

As an E.R. doc, I see every possible health problem. I treat everything from heart attacks to concussions to gunshot wounds and food poisoning. I even treat little kids who think it's a great idea to stuff crayons up their noses.

My patients there—almost all of them—tend to look at what has happened to them and think: *What rotten luck.*

So it was with the guy who came into the E.R. that Saturday night. The lid on his soft drink wasn't on right, so he tried to adjust it—while going 45 miles an hour on the turnpike and eating a fast-food burger. Next thing he knew, his car came to a rest on the median and he was bleeding from multiple wounds, with untold internal damage.

What rotten luck.

My dozen years of medical education and experience tell me that luck has almost nothing to do with it. Our lives are determined by choices we make every day. Should I cook myself a hot breakfast at home, or grab a doughnut at the coffee cart near work? Should I take a walk after dinner, or settle in with the tube? They seem like small decisions at the time, but the difference these choices make is enormous.

I could list for you all the negative consequences of making the wrong choices. But as long as I've got your attention—as long as you're willing to spend the length of this book learning about how to change your life—then I'd much rather point out to you all the positive consequences of taking *The Lean Belly Prescription* to heart.

Among the benefits:

➜ You'll lose weight and look better than ever—as much as 15 pounds in just the next 4 weeks.

➜ You'll enjoy your life more because you'll be free of the pain and hassles extra weight entails. In fact, women who keep their weight within normal range are 40 percent less likely to develop arthritis than obese women.

→ You'll dodge three of the biggest killers out there—heart attacks, diabetes, and stroke—and be much less likely to get cancer.

→ You'll have more energy because your metabolism will be revving high, and you'll have the physical strength to take you places you've never been before.

→ You'll have more money to spend, because people who take care of their bodies look better and earn more money as a result of it—up to 15.4 percent more!

→ You'll be more confident, because you will have demonstrated to yourself that you can tackle something important and succeed.

→ You'll have more and better sex. More sex because obese people who slim down to their ideal weight are considered 43 percent more attractive to the opposite sex; better sex because sexual function is largely about good blood circulation. Less body fat means better blood flow—in all the places you need it.

→ You'll add active years to your life—as much as a decade more to play with the grandkids, travel, watch 3,000 more sunsets and 3,001 more sunrises.

I'll go into all these benefits, and more, in chapter 3. But before I get there I'm asking you to stop right now and take a look at your life, and envision living it the way you want to, for as long as you want to, feeling the way you want to. Can you motor up the stairs rather than pausing after every five for a break? Are your weekends filled with fun activities rather than naps to compensate for your constant exhaustion? Are you still in the game at the office, or are younger and more vigorous people bypassing you?

And, looking off into the future a bit: Will your grandkids remember you as the active grandparent who matched them step for step and showed by example what it really means to be alive? Or will they remember you by your weight or your limitations, and be left with the idea that getting older means getting fatter, weaker, unhealthier?

I believe that *The Lean Belly Prescription* will give you ways to answer each of the upbeat questions with a resounding "yes," and make the negatives vanish. And you'll accomplish those things not by radically altering your daily life, or by giving up the things you love, but by making small changes to your diet and your daily habits, and learning to live lean—for life.

As a doctor, that's the prescription I've always wanted to write.

This book is it.

The Lean Belly Prescription At-A-Glance

This guide summarizes the principles of *The Lean Belly Prescription*: the fast and foolproof diet and weight-loss plan from America's top urgent-care doctor.

Dr. Travis's Eight Laws of Leanness

PICK 3 TO LEAN! Choose any three of the following life-altering dietary changes, and use the law that accompanies it. Depending on your current diet and weight, you could lose up to 15 pounds in 4 weeks, eating foods you love and doing things you enjoy!

- -

1 **If you love cheese and yogurt:** Discover the amazing weight-loss powers of dairy. Eat at least 3 servings of dairy a day, including one at breakfast, and lose up to 3 pounds in 4 weeks!

2 **If you love pasta and rice:** Simply switch all your refined carbs to whole-grain versions, and lose up to 8 pounds in 4 weeks!

3 **If you love soda:** Learn why substituting *more* delicious and refreshing drinks can help you to lose up to 4 pounds in 4 weeks!

4 **If you love to graze:** Nosh all day long on your favorite fruits and vegetables, keep your belly full, and lose up to 6 pounds in 4 weeks!

5 **If you love breakfast:** Build yours around simple lean protein/good carb principles and lose up to 4 pounds in 4 weeks!

6 **If you love to snack:** Learn how to combine food groups to build snacks, and lose up to 7 pounds in 4 weeks!

7 **If you love milk shakes:** Discover how the right milk-shake recipe can help you lose up to 4 pounds in 4 weeks!

8 **If you love to eat fatty foods:** Turn fat into your ally, discover which fats can actually strip away pounds, and lose up to 4 pounds in 4 weeks!

The Lean-Living Turbochargers

Want even faster results? Choose any or all of the following statements and follow the activity plan that accompanies it. It will multiply the effects of your PICK 3 plan *and* make your life more fun.

- -

1 **If you love watching TV:** Pledge to spend 10 minutes on your feet and active—puttering around the house or yard, cooking something delicious from Chapter 5—for every hour you spend watching TV. The average American watches 5 hours a day; cut your average, and you can live lean for life.

2 **If you love spending time with your family:** Spend just 20 minutes a day doing something active with someone you love. It could be as simple as taking a walk, riding bikes, or making whoopie. While you're building stronger family bonds, you'll burn an extra 100 calories a day!

3 **If you love a change of pace:** All you need is one hour a week of "interval training"—a simple workout that involves exercising fast, then exercising slow. Commit to 3 times a week for just 20 minutes! (You'll find the complete program on page 146.)

4 **If you love avoiding exercise:** Yep, there's even a plan for that! It's the magic of non-exercise activity thermogenesis (NEAT), and it means burning calories without breaking a sweat. I'll show you the little tweaks you can make to your daily routine that will start burning fat immediately!

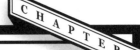

The Promise of Living Lean

Every single day, you face 200 choices that can make the difference between a lifetime of leanness, or a lifetime of troubling trips to the doctor. Here's how to recognize those choices—and banish belly fat for good!

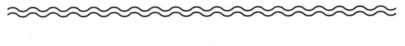

I grew up in the Midwest. My mom was from Iowa, my dad from Nebraska, and I spent my childhood knocking around Missouri, Kansas, and Oklahoma—in the nation's vast middle, you might say.

We were meat-and-potatoes people. Okay, there were vegetables on the table as well, but when the broccoli arrived, it was covered with cheese. Or butter. Or, on really good nights, both. My mom knew she should get us kids to eat our vegetables; she didn't know that drowning them in Velveeta wasn't the best way to do it.

Likewise with my dad, who worked as an animal-feed salesman. He was busy fattening up pigs and cattle, so that meant he was also fattening up the people—including himself—who ate the animals he catered to. There was an all-you-can-eat barbecue joint near his office, and he was one of its best customers. He looked it, too, with a belly that often stalked into the room a second or two before he did.

And that's what I thought "normal" was. (No wonder my favorite breakfast was sausage and peanut butter on an English muffin.)

I never questioned the assumption that belly fat was normal, at least until I left for college, and ended up as an undergraduate at Duke University in Durham, North Carolina. The kids were from all over the country there, and a large part of my education took place outside of the classroom. I can still remember meeting a special subset of the characters in Gilbert-Addoms Hall, my dormitory. They were the "healthy lifestyle" gang. They were the first humans I ever spotted eating yogurt (imagine!), and when their care packages arrived from home, they pulled out cookies made with whole-wheat flour. To a kid from the farmbelt like me, they might as well have been eating cheese straight from the moon. And they exercised—not just by weightlifting or playing sports, like me, but by going on hikes, biking around campus, and walking instead of taking the bus. Fitness was a part of their lifestyles.

I could see it gave them more energy, sharper features, more life.

CHAPTER 1
LAWS OF
LEANNESS

| Belly fat is killer fat, but fortunately it's also the easiest to lose. | Your family and friends are your most important allies in weight loss. |

And I came to a realization: That's what I wanted for my life, as well.

I decided to follow their examples. At first, it wasn't easy: They didn't teach you much about eating well back in my high school, and I made a lot of mistakes. For example, I knew that chicken was a healthy meat, so I started eating lots of fried-chicken sandwiches on giant white rolls, dressed with plenty of cheese and mayo. (Little did I know that, after all the battering and frying and schmearing, I would have been better off eating a hamburger!) It would take me a few years of experimenting to figure out what worked for me, and a few more years of medical school before I fully understood the mechanisms behind weight gain (and weight loss). But as I studied more and more medicine, and learned more about the dangers of belly fat, I started to understand how to make healthy choices in life. I came up with strategies that worked—some gleaned from my medical training, some from my healthy friends, quite a few from unhealthy friends—and the evidence was plain: I was visibly healthier and more energetic. While the guys I went to high school with were growing potbellies by their mid-twenties, I was staying just as lean as I'd been in 12th grade. So people started asking me for advice.

My parents, for instance.

LOOK YOUNGER, FEEL YOUNGER

Now, trying to convince your parents to change their lifestyle isn't easy, even if they're open to what you have to say. At first my parents made just a few changes—taking a walk after dinner, shopping a little smarter—but one good thing led to another for them. Sure, my dad still enjoys his burgers with blue cheese on them (just like his

Less weight around your middle means more energy to live (and love) your life.	Your background isn't a life sentence; you have the power to change.	Losing fat lowers blood pressure and eases pain in your back, legs, and feet.	You make 200 weight-related choices every day. That's 200 chances to start a new life!

son!), but now he snacks on nuts instead of chips, swaps whole-wheat bread for the white stuff, uses a tab of butter rather than the whole tub, and eats more lean chicken and fish than steak—though he still enjoys that occasionally, as well. My parents had been locked into one lifestyle, but they gradually began to feel (and see) the benefits of new approaches that allowed them to eat better, feel better, and live better (and, I hope, live longer at the same time).

Now my dad is 67, and he weighs almost 30 pounds less than he did at the height of his animal-fattening days. He recently visited me in Nashville to help me out with a bunch of home projects—yard work, staining the deck, putting up blinds—going dawn to dusk at my side. I'd dare any 30-year-old to try to keep up with him.

As for my mom, she's so accustomed to her new, healthful ways of cooking and eating that she's forgotten that the Velveeta era ever happened. Her healthful way of life now seems so natural to her that she can't imagine living any other way. One of the many rewards: She looks at least a decade younger than her age, which I've promised never to disclose. (You owe me, Mom!)

How did they reach their current healthy states? They made smart, incremental moves for the better, and they were able to enjoy the benefits of their new lifestyle as they went along. So in a way, they were the first success stories from *The Lean Belly Prescription*. The strategies outlined in this book have worked for me. They've worked for my friends, my family, and later, my patients. And science proves that they will work for you, too!

WHY BELLY FAT IS AN EMERGENCY

If you're carrying extra weight in your abdomen, you'd probably admit that it looks pretty unsightly on the outside. Well, it looks even worse on the inside. I know, because I've seen it there.

Many times, sick or injured patients come under my care soon after they've eaten an excessively fatty meal. How do I know? I can literally spot the fat globules that are swimming in their blood, just like an oil slick from a broken drilling platform. More times than not, those globules help explain why these unfortunate folks are in the E.R. in the first place. Bloodborne fat blobs are like homing pigeons, looking to roost in the body's fat cells. And unless a famine breaks out, that's right where they'll stay.

There are serious health implications to that, for both men and women. Men are most likely to pack excess fat around their internal organs, which is known as visceral fat. (Ladies, that can happen to you, too, though you're more likely to pack it in your legs, arms, and butt. That's no picnic, either. After menopause, though, you'll be more likely to gain weight in the gut, too.) You know you have visceral fat if your gut is round and firm, your waist is bigger than your hips, or your Wranglers have a waist size of 40 or higher for men, and 35 or higher for women. If that description fits you, it probably means your body is storing your excess fat like packing peanuts that surround and infiltrate your muscles, heart, liver, kidneys, intestines, and pancreas.

But visceral fat doesn't just lie there, looking ugly. It actively works to harm your body by secreting a number of substances, collectively called adipokines. Adipokines include a hormone called resistin, which leads to high blood sugar and raises your risk of diabetes; angiotensinogen, a compound that raises blood pressure; and interleukin-6, a chemical associated with arterial inflammation and heart disease. Visceral fat also messes with another important hormone called adiponectin, which regulates the metabolism of lipids and glucose. The more belly fat you have, the less adiponectin you have, and the lower your metabolism. (And here's the crazy part: The lower your metabolism, the more belly fat you'll store. It's as though belly fat is conspiring to harm you by breeding even more belly fat!)

Meanwhile your liver, faced with a high tide of fat globules, feels like it's swimming in energy. But as it burns that overly abundant energy source, it produces excess cholesterol, which in turn gunks up your arteries in the form of plaque. Allow that plaque buildup to continue for a decade or more, and that's when you and I will meet in the E.R.; your increased risks of stroke, heart attack, and diabetes will pay off in an "event."

But just because it's more business for my shop doesn't mean I'll be particularly happy to see you there in that condition. As I said in the introduction to this book, the most frustrating part of my job as a doctor is having to treat people who are a long way down a road they never should have taken in the first place. The more belly fat you carry, the greater your risk for any number of health worries. And the greater your health risks, the more you're going to find your medicine cabinet filled with little brown prescription bottles. In the medical journal *BMC Family Practice*, I saw a chart showing that people with body mass indexes of 30 or higher took up to twice as many prescription drugs as those whose BMIs were less than 25. In fact, overweight people spend 37 percent more money at the pharmacy each year than people of desirable weight; once you reach the level of obesity, your prescription medical costs are an average of 105 percent higher than those of normal-weight folks! That's a burden on not just your checkbook, but also your health in general.

Here's how the problem starts building. For starters, if you're carrying too much weight in your belly, it's probably putting a lot of strain on your back, legs, and joints, so you might be on a pain med. But pain meds often produce constipation, so maybe you get a stool softener, too.

COMPARED WITH OBESE WOMEN,

WOMEN *with* LEAN BELLIES ARE...

57%
less likely to
die of heart disease

40%
less likely to
die of cancer

12%
less likely to
have a stroke

40%
less likely to
develop arthritis of the
hips or knees

69%
less likely to
develop type 2 diabetes

21%
less likely to experience
arousal dysfunction

Your cholesterol is likely high, so perhaps you've had a statin thrown into the mix, along with the blood pressure meds that come with all of those extra miles of blood vessels and capillaries needed to service your added bulk. Heavy people are more likely to be diabetic, so you might be on any number of pills or injections designed to keep your blood sugar in check. But your circulation might be out of whack, too, so maybe that's brought on the blood thinners that can help you avoid a stroke or heart attack. And the guys who are just looking for a little love (to help them forget all of the above) may have to pop a little blue pill to help them boost blood flow where they need it, to please themselves and the missus. Being overweight adds to sleep disturbances, so toss the occasional sleeping pill into the mix. Obese people are also 50 percent more likely to suffer from asthma (more meds), 150 percent more likely to develop gallstones (still more meds), and are more prone to depression than the general population (even more meds!).

You see the point I'm making: What begins as a weight problem can quickly accelerate through many other body systems. And rather than address the root cause—the weight—people tend to ask for another drug as a quick fix.

And that's why belly fat isn't just an unsightly annoyance. It's a real health emergency.

Good thing you've got an urgent-care doctor on call!

SMALL CHANGES LEAD TO A DRAMATICALLY BETTER LIFE

If you've struggled with weight issues for a long time, or if you've grown frustrated with your inability to control weight gain, you might look at your belly and see a problem you simply can't beat, no matter how big a life change you're willing to make. And quite frankly, you're right. No one has ever climbed a mountain in one giant step. What it takes is a series of small steps, one after the other, until you look around and say, "Holy cow! I'm on top of the world!"

And what's great is that even small steps, once you take them, can make an enormous impact on your looks, your health, and your life. For example, the folks who ran a UK study called the Counterweight Programme looked at the impact of a 10 percent weight change. The math major in me looks at 10 percent and says: Now that's possible. If you're laboring under a 220-pound load, getting down to a solid 198 can deliver a whole new world for you.

Take a look at these eye-popping stats. If an obese person loses 10 percent of his or her weight, it will result in a:

31 percent decrease in risk of diabetes

20 percent decrease in risk of high blood-fat levels

25 percent decrease in risk of high blood pressure

21 percent decrease in risk of cardiovascular disease (which includes coronary heart disease, myocardial infarction, congestive heart failure, stroke, and transient ischemic attack)

I love numbers, so I'm a sucker for those percentage drops in risk. The bottom line is that you don't have to get all the way to super-model slim to enjoy enormous physical, financial, and emotional benefits. If you manage to meet this highly doable level of weight loss, you're potentially saving yourself years of backless-gown

COMPARED WITH OBESE MEN,

MEN *with* LEAN BELLIES ARE...

32%
less likely to
die of heart disease

45%
less likely to
develop cancer

60%
less likely to
develop arthritis

83%
less likely to
develop diabetes

32%
less likely to
develop sleep apnea

61%
less likely to have
erectile dysfunction

embarrassment, waiting-room boredom, and possibly even pulse-pounding terror in the ambulance. And the lower your weight goes beyond that initial 10 percent drop, the lower your risk goes, as well. So we're not talking about cruel blows of fate, but rather *variables you have within your power to control.*

The power to live leaner. To live healthier. To live longer. In fact, a 2009 study published in *The Lancet* showed that normal-weight people could expect to live as much as 10 years longer than people who are morbidly obese. *That's an entire decade* to get to know your grand-kids or walk on the beach with your husband or wife. Another decade to make plans and realize them. More retirement, less work!

If altering the number on your scale can tip so many other numbers in your favor, why wouldn't you do it? Because you don't want to "go on a diet"?

Heh, heh. Good. Because I don't want you to go on a diet, either!

TINY CHANGES, BIG RESULTS

Please note that I didn't put the word "diet" in the title of this book. That's because my prescription refers to the food and activity choices we make, not to a restrictive eating plan. I did that for a good reason: Going after weight gain by going on a diet is like walking into a gun-fight with a sharp stick. You might make a little dent, but in the end, you'll do yourself more harm than good.

Here's why: Typical diets restrict calories, and that means lowering your metabolism—the calorie furnace in your body that determines longterm weight loss. Going on a diet sends a signal to your body that says "I'm starving here!" And your body responds by slowing your metabolic rate in order to hold on to existing energy stores. What's worse, if the food shortage (meaning your crash diet) continues, you'll begin burning muscle tissue, which just gives your enemy, visceral fat, a greater advantage. Your metabolism drops even more, and fat goes on to claim even more territory. That's why my PICK 3 TO LEAN plan doesn't involve cutting calories drastically—it merely helps you swap out nutritionally empty food and replace it with healthier versions of the same foods you enjoy now.

Want proof that you can lose substantial amounts of weight—and keep it off for good—without ever dieting? Cutting-edge research that I pulled together to write this book points the way to quick and easy weight loss. For example:

1 Muscle Up Your Metabolism

Quite simply, metabolism is the rate at which our bodies burn the energy from food calories. During your skinny teens, your body was a raging, hormonally fed inferno. But your burn rate falls by 2 percent every 10 years from your twenties onward, and you know what happens to energy that isn't used: It's stored as fat.

➡ *Muscle is several times more metabolically active than fat. The more muscle you have, the hotter your fire burns. And if you activate those muscles through physical activity, the potential fat burn can last for up to 24 hours. Any light exercise that maintains muscle mass will attack fat at the same time.*

the KEYS TO LOSING

To determine the most effective lifestyle strategies for losing weight, researchers at the Centers for Disease Control and Prevention surveyed nearly 600 successful "losers" on their efforts. Here's what they found.

71%	47%	36%	19%	10%
Ate more fruits and vegetables	Exercised at least 30 minutes a day	Planned meals	Lifted weights	Jogged or ran

People who skipped workouts due to "lack of time" were 76 percent less likely to maintain their weight loss.

2 Help Your Loved Ones Lose Weight

One of the more fascinating pieces of obesity-related research I've read came out in the *New England Journal of Medicine* in 2007. Researchers looked at data on 12,000 people—many of them related to one another—who'd been tracked in the Framingham Heart Study. Their conclusion: A person was at greater risk for being obese if others in his or her social network were obese. The stats: If a friend became obese, risk climbed by 57 percent; if a sibling became obese, risk went up by 40 percent; a spouse, plus 37 percent.

➡ *The same study concluded that the benefits of weight loss may radiate through social networks as well. So if you share this book with friends and family, you'll all have a better chance of realizing its benefits. And think about how cool it will be around the Thanksgiving table next year, when you all look awesome! Pass the brussels sprouts!*

3 Make the Most of Your Morning

A study from the University of Massachusetts Medical School determined that people who skip breakfast are 4½ times more likely to be obese than people who make time for it. An expert from the University of Pittsburgh Medical Center estimated that going without breakfast can slow your metabolism by up to 10 percent.

➡ *Build breakfast out of protein and healthy fat. Eggs. Greek yogurt. Peanut butter. Milk. The more protein you eat, the more satisfied you'll be: A 2008 study published in the* **British Journal of Nutrition** *noted that the protein can lead to feelings of fullness that last all day long.*

4 Sip Your Way Slim

You're made out of water—over 60 percent, by most reckonings. So you need to drink plenty of it. But talk about Trojan horses: In the past 30 years, we've more than doubled the number of calories we drink, raising it to 450 on average today. Why? Because we stopped drinking water, and started drinking sugar water!

➡ *If you take only one thing from this chapter, make it this: If a drink has added sugar, it's liquid fat. Bottled blubber. Fizzy flab. Drinkable derriere. Caboose in a can. Phase it out of your drinking diet, and you'll make huge strides toward shedding unwelcome, unnecessary weight. The strategy on page 64 can get you started.*

5 Stop Being Harassed by Clowns

A study from Yale University's Rudd Center for Food Policy and Obesity found that 50 percent of kids said the food in a box with Shrek's green mug on it tasted better than the very same food in a Shrekless box. And what kinds of food most often have cartoon characters on them? Right: sugar-laden ones. Adults fall prey to similar marketing techniques on their foods' packaging as well. But guess what? An apple doesn't come with a label.

➡ *Beware packaged foods that present you with meaningless buzzwords like "natural," "fat free," "diet," and "a smart choice"—and ingredient lists longer than Al Capone's rap sheet. When you buy whole foods as they grew in nature—a salmon fillet, green beans, an orange—each has only one ingredient: the food itself. All of your grocery store transactions should be so simple.*

6 Shrink Your Pot, Shrink Your Belly

I kid you not. Brian Wansink, Ph.D., a food visionary who runs the Cornell University Food and Brand Lab, has devoted extraordinary attention to the effects that the containers that carry our food and drink have on how much we consume. His rule of thumb: The larger the plate or bowl or glass, the more you will eat or slurp or drink from it. The bad news: We're on the wrong side of a century-long expansion in the sizes of our dinner plates and the volumes of our drinking glasses. As go your portion sizes, so goes your personal size.

➡ *Instead of 1 cup of chocolate ice cream, enjoy ½ cup of chocolate ice cream with ½ cup of sliced strawberries. The fruit tastes great, adds tons of antioxidants, and saves you 115 calories.*

These are exactly the kind of small changes you can make that will have an enormous impact on your future. Indeed, people who struggle with weight issues don't need to completely make over their lifestyles to completely make over their lives. The very latest research and most cutting-edge science—the expertise that informs *The Lean Belly Prescription*—shows that it's the small changes that make the biggest difference.

200 CHANCES TO
LOSE WEIGHT TODAY

In 2007, the medical journal *Environment and Behavior* ran a study showing that on an average day, we average people are faced with more than 200 choices that have an impact on our weight:

• Breakfast at home, on the road, or not at all?
• Fries with that?
• Cheese on those fries?
• Small, medium, large, extra large, or Big Gulp?

These choices play into the question of whether we'll continue to wear the 44-inch jeans that feel comfortable now, or whether we can return to the 32-inch waistbands we wore back in college. That's 200 chances every day to become fatter, sicker, less happy— or 200 opportunities every day to choose the right foods that bring us leanness, health, and joy. Two hundred opportunities to fight belly fat and the negative health outcomes that come with it. Two hundred opportunities to look better in our clothes (and out of them), to be more energetic, and to feel better about ourselves. And given the way weight impacts social and family circles, it's also 200 opportunities to be a positive influence on the lives of the people we love most.

I've told the story about how that dynamic has worked in my own family, spreading to my mom and dad and close friends. Now I'm redrawing my circle to include you among the people whose lives I want to change for the better.

So here's my pledge to you: I'll go every step of the way with you, I'll be realistic about your prospects, and I'll only propose strategies I know will work. I'll give you a whole selection of easy, life-altering changes you can make to your daily diet, and I'll only ask you to make three of them—PICK 3 TO LEAN! And then I'll give you four of the world's easiest fat-burning strategies, and yep, you only have to pick one of those, too!

Your reward is this: an energetic new life in which good health is an investment that pays off for years to come. In place of all those expensive prescription drugs at the pharmacy, you'll have something priceless: a *Lean Belly Prescription* that can help you make better choices every minute of every day and free you to live the life you want.

10 SECOND SLIMDOWN | Better Health

Your weight may be the single most important influence on your health over the years ahead. Invest 10 seconds now, and save yourself decades of trouble later.

RUIN YOUR APPETITE

Consuming a liquid to begin a meal can reduce your total calorie intake by up to 20 percent because it makes you feel full. To avoid having to pound two glasses of H$_2$O, try this: Drink one glass and start with a broth-based soup, like miso, minestrone, or chicken noodle.

SIGN UP FOR A RACE

If you find a better reason to work out than pure weight loss, you'll be more likely to maintain an exercise program, says a University of Michigan study. Find an event at active.com.

BE REALISTIC

The key to diet longevity is a realistic, flexible eating plan, says Alan Aragon, M.S., a nutritionist in Thousand Oaks, California. Most people eat too little and go into defensive mode when cravings strike. Then they cheat, then feel bad, then resist, and then cheat again. It's an endless cycle. If you're craving Häagen-Dazs, grab a spoon. Just dig in moderation.

IGNITE YOUR FAT BURNERS

Capsaicin, the compound that gives chile peppers their mouth-searing quality, can also fire up your metabolism, according to a study in the *Journal of Nutritional Science and Vitaminology*. Eat about 1 tablespoon of chopped red or green chiles to boost your body's production of heat and the activity of your sympathetic nervous system. The result is a metabolism spike of 23 percent!

ELIMINATE ADDED SUGARS

According to a USDA survey, the average American eats about 20 teaspoons of added sugar daily, or 317 empty calories. The researchers report that 82 percent of that added sugar can be attributed to soda, baked goods, breakfast cereals, candy, and fruit drinks. What's not on the list? Meat, vegetables, whole fruit, and eggs, along with unsweetened whole-grain and dairy products. Eat accordingly.

SCRAMBLE TO SLIM DOWN

Not only are eggs a great muscle-building food, but they can also help you look less egg-shaped. A 2010 study in *Nutrition Research* showed that men who had eggs for breakfast ate less over the next 24 hours than those who began their day with a bagel instead. (The cholesterol in eggs isn't a heart threat; cancel the egg-white omelets!)

SET GOOD GOALS
University of Iowa scientists found that people who monitored their diet and exercise goals most frequently were more likely to achieve them than were goal setters who rarely reviewed their objectives.

SPICE THINGS UP
Ground cinnamon has been shown to help prevent insulin resistance, which means it may slow the sugar in frozen yogurt from passing through your stomach too quickly, thus suppressing the blood-sugar spike. Sprinkle some atop your next cone or cup.

STRIKE OUT OVEREATING

If you skimp all day before eating out, you'll be so hungry that you end up overdoing it. Instead, eat a healthy snack that contains protein and fiber a few hours before your meal. Fat-free yogurt or a small bowl of whole-grain cereal with low-fat milk are smart choices.

PRACTICE MIND OVER MUNCHIES

Tempted to dive headfirst into your plate when you feel stressed? Try this: Visualize your negative thoughts riding by on a conveyor belt. Label each one ("Big project due at work!" or "First-date jitters!"), then imagine it chugging into oblivion. Research subjects at Temple University's Center for Obesity Research and Education say this method has helped them avoid emotional eating.

CHAPTER 2

All Your Weight Worries—
Solved!

Afraid you can't lose weight and keep it off for good? There's an answer for every concern— and a plan to overcome every excuse!

~~~~~~

S aving lives is something I do for a living. But it was a life we saved on the set of *The Doctors* that still resonates as one of my proudest moments. We performed a weight-loss intervention on a crew member: my friend Chunky B.

Chunky B is a comedian by trade, and his job was to warm up the studio audience. So before my colleagues and I would take the stage, Chunky B would be out there cracking up the audience and getting them psyched for our arrival. He was as critical to the show's early success as anyone else on the team. To look at him now, lean and fit, he's the kind of guy you'd look at and think, "Lucky bum, he's never had a weight problem in his whole life."

Well, you'd be wrong.

When I was getting to know him during the premiere season of *The Doctors,* he was the lovable fat guy who audiences enjoyed laughing with. The problem: They laughed *at* him, too. His weight—263 pounds at the time—was good comedy material. (Classic line: "My wife had the nerve to say, 'Chunky, you need to get in shape.' I looked straight at her and said, 'Honey, round *is* a shape.'") Being chubby means being vulnerable, and a soft underbelly is kind of funny on a guy, right? But while the extra pounds were earning him laughs, they were secretly ruining every other aspect of his life.

At one point during that first season, Chunky B took me aside and made a brief confession—nothing funny about it. "Travis," he told me, "I spend all day listening to you talk about health, and I'm scared. I'm overweight, tired all the time, and I don't feel good. I don't even have the energy to play with my kids. I need help."

The sad truth was that he hadn't always been Chunky B, and now he considered his nickname—and his funny-fat-guy identity—a burden. He'd been an athlete in college, playing soccer and revving like a toddler on Mountain Dew. But over time, the same thing happened to him that has happened to two out of every three Americans: He traded daily exercise for sofa surfing, his muscle mass and daily calorie burn plunged, and yet he kept eating as if he were still a

CHAPTER
2

LAWS OF
LEANNESS

83% of people who lose flab and keep it off can trace their weight loss to a single moment of truth.

Photographs can expose lies—even white ones—you may be telling yourself about your weight.

19-year-old soccer star. He packed on the pounds. He was like Wile E. Coyote chasing that roadrunner straight off the cliff. For a moment, he could run straight ahead on nothing but the air, but before long gravity—and his extra flab—dragged him down.

As we noted in the last chapter, your metabolism is the rate at which your body burns fuel. Everything from breathing to maintaining your heartbeat to digesting dinner requires energy, as does the more obvious stuff like shoveling snow, taking a walk, and chasing the grandkids. The more fuel you burn, the less fat you carry around. But unfortunately, your metabolism slows down both as you gain weight *and* as you grow older.

When you're gaining weight, your flagging metabolism is like the force of gravity that pulled the poor coyote to the bottom of the cliff. Unless you exercise regularly, your body starts to go soft as you age—and sooner than you think. For every year after you turn 25, you lose 1 percent of your muscle. That's no tragedy when you go from 100 percent stoked at age 25 to 99 percent at 26, but the real shocker arrives at age 40, when you're left with only 85 percent of a shrinking inventory of muscle. Guess what shows up to fill the empty shelves at Warehouse You? Belly fat.

At the time Chunky B confided in me, he didn't know any of this. He just knew he didn't feel well and that he was sick of being thought of as a funny overweight guy. Being merely funny—and much healthier and happier—would be a breakthrough for him.

So we did an intervention right on the show. We ran Chunky B through a series of medical tests, and then I called him onstage and revealed his vital stats to the world. But more important, I revealed them to *him*. And they were terrifying:

• **Blood pressure:** 170/100 (anything above 120/80 puts you at

Losing just 10% of your body weight will have profound effects.	Going on a diet is another way of saying "going to fail."	You can burn calories without ever lifting a weight or running a mile.	A slowing metabolism means you're gaining more weight eating the same food.

increased risk of heart attack and stroke)

- **Weight:** 263 pounds
- **Total cholesterol:** 183
- **Body fat percentage:** 29

Upon hearing his numbers, he knew exactly why he felt the way he did. He was literally being weighed down by years of bad choices on food, exercise, and lifestyle. He was a success in his chosen field but felt miserable inside. At age 44, he was at the proverbial crossroads, and I could tell him where taking the straight path would lead: straight off Coyote Cliff. Under the glare of the lights and with an audience of millions watching, I asked him if he was really ready to lose the weight. He didn't hesitate: "I'm committed, 100 percent."

And soon, a new man was born. The transformation was remarkable. Within 6 weeks, he had dropped nearly 20 pounds. And 6 months later, we brought the former Chunky B back on stage to reveal his new body, and a new nickname I coined: Hunky B. Here's the tale of the tape:

- **Blood pressure:** 126/80
- **Weight:** 223
- **Total cholesterol:** 131
- **Body fat percentage:** 22

How did he get there?

Not by going on a fad diet.

Not by spending hours in the gym each day.

Not by giving up the things he loved to eat.

Not by feeling hungry, deprived, or miserable.

Instead, he simply followed the easy, sensible advice you'll find in *The Lean Belly Prescription*. He chose the nutrition and lifestyle changes that suited his time, his tastes, and his goals. He learned enough about nutrition to guide him safely through the eating decisions he needed to make every day. (Chapter 4 will help you do the same.) He found ways to incorporate non-exercise calorie burning into his day to help augment his 44-year-old metabolism. (Chapter 6 has an exercise plan for you that's unlike any other you've ever tried.)

But most important of all, he made the decision that all that body fat he was carrying wasn't really *him*. And this is an important point I want to drive home: You may be fat, but that fat is not you. It is an alien invader inside your body, trying to cause you harm. And you need to fight back.

YOUR SUCCESS STORY BEGINS NOW!

People who lose weight and keep it off—like my pal Chunky B—often have a body fat epiphany: a moment of truth when they realize that they're too heavy and need to lose weight—or else. The National Weight Control Registry catalogued those moments by the percentage of participants who reported them:

22.9%
cited medical triggers,
like when a doctor informed them of the consequences of being overweight. (Wait no longer: I'm a doctor, and I'm informing you!)

21.3%
cited breaking their own weight record,
a kind of lifetime high point that nobody wants to see.

12.7%
saw an unflatteringly pudgy picture of themselves
or a reflection of themselves in what they first thought was a fun-house mirror—but no such luck.

8.7%
found the will to lose when they started a new job
or were approaching their 40th birthday. (Another reason to accept the invite to the high-school reunion!)

6.9%
were motivated by an embarrassing moment,
like when a co-worker teased them about their weight.

5.3%
said it happened when they found a weight-loss program they liked.
(I hope this one does the trick for you.)

5%
were inspired by a weight-loss success story,
like when they watched Oprah fit into smaller jeans, or when a friend shared his or her own weight-loss secret.

My favorite thing about this list:
So many of the moments were positive ones. I hope, if you haven't found yours, it's waiting for you in these pages.

FIND YOUR WEIGHT-LOSS SPARK—AND BURN AWAY FLAB FOREVER!

I wish I could do the same thing for all 160 million overweight American adults as I did for Chunky—sorry, I mean Hunky—B. But 160 million, that's a lot of people to try to fit onto one show. The green room—where guests wait before they join us onstage—only holds about eight people! Think how much coffee they'd drink—and the line at the bathroom!

So if you're game, I'll do the intervention right here, between the covers of this book. The upside: Our viewers across the country won't know your body fat percentage. And we can enjoy a doctor-patient privilege similar to the one you get in an examination room. Let's start with the most troublesome part of your body, where weight gain starts.

I'm talking about your brain.

It turns out that Chunky B's moment of truth isn't an unusual thing in the world of weight-loss success stories. The study from the National Weight Control Registry showed that more than 83 percent of successful dieters remembered a single emotional or physical incident that helped them turn the corner toward skinny. And they didn't have to hear their weight stats broadcast around the country to do it.

It could have been a dad who suddenly found himself too winded to continue chasing his toddler through the playground.

It could have been a woman who turned down an invite from a friend to join the charity bike ride because she wasn't sure she could do it anymore.

It could have been a 45-year-old man who received a panicked phone call from his mother saying that his dad had been admitted to the hospital with chest pains.

It could have been a 35-year-old looks at her niece's wedding photos on Facebook and initially doesn't recognize the heavy-set person wearing her dress.

It could be you when your invitation arrives for your 15th high-school reunion and you wonder how you'll look to your classmates.

Or when you hear your doctor's murmured worry about your blood sugar readings that are consistently coming in too high.

Or when you contemplate whether to donate your favorite jeans (which you haven't fit into in this century) to charity.

Or when back pain joins foot pain and knee pain on your list of why you can't possibly begin an exercise program or even walk comfortably from the car into the mall.

Or it could be a bit of personal illumination that comes when the light shines out as you open the fridge at 1 a.m.

All of these moments can be painful ones—physically painful, and emotionally painful. I clearly remember the stunned silence on the set of *The Doctors* when everyone could see that Chunky B, for once, was no longer laughing.

Maybe you're in the same position when it comes to your belly fat—laughing about it on the outside, but embarrassed, worried, maybe even a little scared on the inside. That's why I want you to have your Chunky B moment right now.

So I'm going to propose an exercise to you. (Don't worry, it doesn't involve a chin-up bar.) Next time you're home on a lazy weekend, take a break and root around in some old photo albums. See if you can piece together a succession of photos of yourself that start at about age 16 and march year by year to the present day. (Recruit Mom if you need help; they're our world's photo archivists, after all.) It's actually pretty fun to follow the time-lapse photography through the different hairstyles, clothing cuts, and people surrounding you. Take a moment to enjoy the nostalgia and laugh at what your husband or wife is wearing in the photos. What was everyone thinking?!

Okay, the fun's over. Now watch your weight as you go along. Is your face growing rounder? Are your clothes cut a little looser? Maybe you can spot the point where the trim beltline of those size-32 jeans gives way to an elastic waistband. The smiles are still bright, but where does the jawline lose a little definition?

If I were looking over your shoulder, I'd be aware of another progression taking place below the surface. As your body shape changes, you're changing inside, too. Cholesterol and plaque are building up in your arteries, triglycerides are storming through your bloodstream, and visceral fat is cozying up to—and threatening—your internal organs. The extra weight is bearing down on every vertebra, but especially on those in your lower back. Women who carry extra weight in their arms and breasts are being pulled forward and are even more at risk for strains. Your lungs are working overtime to oxygenate the extra blood you're pumping to supply your bigger body, and your heart is like the central water station in Houston on the hottest day of the year, working at max capacity to send fluids to distant suburbs. It's all physical stress on your most important bodily systems—and it's impossible to sustain for long without a breakdown.

Now I'll fan the photos forward in time, projecting the images along two different life paths—only one of which you'll enjoy.

First, the dark side: More years and Thanksgiving dinners pass, and more pie wedges vanish. If your belly-fat-accumulating lifestyle continues unchecked, more physical transformations may occur. Your blood pressure will probably creep up into the danger zone as your blood sugar rises. Your skeleton and connective tissues will buckle under the strain of carrying more weight than they're designed for, and you'll develop physical pains that will severely limit what you can do in life. You'll tell your daughter to take the grandkids to Disney without you and just send you a postcard if they think of it. Then comes the big one: Years of taking in too many refined carbohydrates will begin to raise your blood sugar even higher. Your pancreas, which has spent years pumping out insulin to manage an overload of sugars in your diet, will begin to grow exhausted, sending you from prediabetes to full-blown diabetes. Not too long afterward, the photo record will cease entirely, because the effects of diabetes can be so devastating.

But enough of that. I prefer looking at the pictures in your brighter future collection.

Here's my hope once you, like Chunky B, fully commit to a lean lifestyle. Four weeks from now, you'll have lost 10, even 15 pounds of flab. Six months from now, you'll have lost more than 10 percent of your body weight. If initially you were a 180-pound woman, you'll be in fighting trim at 162 pounds. Because abdominal fat is both the easiest to put on and the easiest to lose, you'll be noticeably thinner around the middle. Your arteries will be in self-cleaning mode as you send less cholesterol and fewer triglycerides through your system. You know how your car performs when you upgrade to high-test? That's what you'll have going when you drop those 15 to 20 pounds. You'll treat your pancreas to a well-deserved trip to Disney because your grandkids feel they need to introduce you to Goofy. (As if the two of you haven't been married for years.)

You'll be in a new wardrobe (you can roll your savings on prescription drugs into your clothing budget), and you'll have more energy than you did a decade ago. **You'll be sleeping better**—and maybe enjoying a little more nonsleep activity in bed as well, because you'll look the part of the romantic lead rather than the romantic ruin. **You'll have more fun.** When your teenagers are shooting baskets, **you'll be free to play** with them without huffing and blowing like a walrus stranded at low tide. **Your standing will be elevated at the office**, because people who take care of themselves always have the edge in pay and promotions. **You won't shy away from the camera** because you'll be eager to paste the next photograph into the line of images—the one that shows you've taken control of your life by taking control of your weight.

If you've now had your "realization moment" à la Chunky B and you're ready to commit to the second scenario, congratulations: I'm with you all the way. One of the best ways to start *The Lean Belly Prescription*, and stick with it, is to make a public declaration of your intentions. You can do that by going to LeanBellyRx.com and making your statement, posting photographs, and sending out notes to family and friends. You'll need them on your side. We've prepared a series of e-mails and newsletters that will help them help you, and maybe they'll pick up some get-skinny suggestions as well.

Now, I know that you've heard all sorts of weight-loss promises in the past—heck, you can't turn on daytime TV without seeing dozens of ads for diet plans, fitness gimmicks, and weight-loss clubs. And chances are, if you've ever tried one of those plans—or if you've considered them, only to shy away out of a fear of failure—then now's the time to stop and confront your fears head on.

We've already talked about the reasons you should try to lose weight. Now, let's talk about the reasons you might avoid trying to lose weight—the most common worries and excuses—and let's knock them down, one by one.

I JUST CAN'T LIVE WITHOUT MY FAVORITE FOODS!

Who's asking you to do that? You're trapped in the old diet-think that demands you give up everything you love most and switch over to all celery, all the time.

In fact, the PICK 3 TO LEAN plan allows you to customize your daily food plan to include your favorite foods! If you love carbs, pick the carb lover's option. If you're a fan of hearty breakfasts, or snacks, or even fatty foods, well, there's a plan for you, too. In fact, all you have to do is simply pick three of your favorite types of foods and commit to eating more of them—yes, that's right, you pick your favorite foods and, with a few small tweaks, you eat more of them. That's worry number one, solved!

➡ *On the PICK 3 TO LEAN plan, you'll be learning so much about the best ways to eat your favorite foods that you'll find you're enjoying them even more. (You'll find the program fully explained in Chapters 4 and 5.)*

I'VE FAILED AT DIETS BEFORE. WHAT MAKES THIS ONE DIFFERENT?

No problem. You can't fail at this diet for one simple reason: This isn't a diet.

A diet is about denying yourself specific foods or limiting yourself to specific calorie counts. It's *not* about listening to what your body needs and enjoys. *The Lean Belly Prescription*, on the other hand, is built on nutritional and psychological science, and it will teach you to listen to your body and its needs more closely than ever and eat more often, not less.

Wait: Eat more often? How can I promise that?

Having an empty belly means a starved brain is calling the shots. Its marching orders at that point: Eat everything, in quantity. If you keep your belly satisfied, the message your brain gets is: Life is good; carry on. You'll be able to bypass the vending machines on your way to work, for the simple reason that you just ate—and oh yes, you're about to eat again!

That's why any weight-loss plan that involves calorie counting is destined to fail. Since when can a number tell you when to stop eating? How much better it is to let your natural bodily systems put on the brakes. And that's just what will happen if you balance fat, fiber, nutrition, and enjoyment in your daily meal plan. To do that, you'll need to build a flavor portfolio that satisfies your needs and makes eating a joy. Then, the awesome foods you've selected will crowd out the junk that's making you fat now and clouding your future later.

➤ *Eating at least five times a day—three well-balanced meals and at least two small, sensible snacks—is critical to keeping your belly and your brain satisfied.*

I HATE RUNNING AND GOING TO THE GYM. CAN I STILL LOSE WEIGHT?

Yes! Just as I take exception to the idea of dieting, I worry about formal exercise plans, too. They're great for people who like them, but they also leave out a great number of us who are too intimidated to begin exercising at a gym. Plus, as with diets, if you go on a workout plan, it's easy to fall off it. So, fine, avoid them at all costs.

How do you feel about walking around the block with your spouse instead? Could you walk down the hall to talk with a co-worker instead of sending an e-mail? Could you plant a garden, volunteer for Habitat for Humanity, participate in the community cleanup day? If so, you can take advantage of a neat little weight-loss secret called, well, NEAT: non-exercise activity thermogenesis. It's essentially a series of small tweaks to your daily life that allows you to ratchet up your calorie burn without engaging in formal exercise.

I know your first thought: Surely just walking around the block isn't enough to change my body! But you're wrong. A study from the Mayo Clinic concluded that the difference between being at a healthy weight and being obese can be as little as *100 calories a day*. You can do that without coming into contact with the no-neck monsters at the Muscle Palace. And I promise that every calorie you burn can be fun and rewarding. Think of it as recess, not a workout!

➤ *Physical activity—of any kind—helps you stick to a healthy eating plan. Researchers at the University of Pittsburgh studied overweight adults and found that one good habit supports the other. I've incorporated that thinking into the activity plans I offer to turbocharge the PICK 3 TO LEAN food plan. The amount of just-plain-movement in your day—walking, doing chores, getting off your duff in general—*

can have a huge impact on the number of calories you burn every day. As much as 2,000 calories a day, according to one study. Tap into that advantage, and you'll never need to visit a gym. Your whole day will be an exercise session, and you'll burn fat 24/7.

I'M WORRIED THAT 6 MONTHS FROM NOW I'M GOING TO START REGAINING THE WEIGHT.

Here's the simple rule of diets: Most diets work in the short term. Most diets fail in the long term. Period. You only need to fear rebound weight gain if you "go on a diet," because at some point you'll "go off" that diet. That's why this isn't a diet plan at all.

Instead, it's a plan that empowers you to eat your favorite foods and engage in your favorite activities—foods and activities so satisfying you wouldn't give them up if laws were passed against them. You'll be enjoying the process so much—and be so eager to share it with your friends and family—that you'll come to think of your new habits as "the way we live now" rather than Dr. Travis's *Lean Belly Prescription*. And you'll find your stresses and worries beginning to dissolve.

➡ *People who engage in physical activity at any intensity for just 17 minutes a day are 61 percent less likely to feel highly stressed than sedentary people, according to researchers in Denmark.*

I JUST DON'T KNOW IF I HAVE THE WILLPOWER!

This isn't a worry, it's a reality. You *may not* have the willpower, period. But then again, neither do I, and probably neither do any of the lean, fit, active people you admire. Willpower is overrated. If it comes down to a test of wills, you may eventually fail.

Make Room for Nature's Perfect Foods

SHRINK YOUR BELLY, BOOST YOUR HEALTH,
AND PLEASE YOUR PALATE WITH THESE ESSENTIAL EATS

The supermarket's a crazy place. You can go cross-eyed comparing labels and decoding ingredient lists. Here, I've handpicked five foods that should make it onto your shopping list every time.

Nuts

WHY THEY'RE HEALTHY: They help you build muscle, fight food cravings, and decrease your risks of obesity, heart disease, and cancer.

HOW TO EAT THEM: With their skins intact, dry roasted, without salt. Keep them handy as a snack: I recommend 2 ounces (two handfuls) of nuts each day.

BEST BETS: almonds, pistachios, cashews

Milk

WHY IT'S HEALTHY: Milk builds strong bones, aids muscle growth, and helps fuel weight loss. It can also help prevent osteoporosis and high blood pressure.

HOW TO DRINK IT: Drink two or three glasses of milk a day and you'll lower your likelihood of both heart attack and stroke, say British scientists.

BEST BETS: 2% milk. It has all the flavor of whole milk, with fewer calories.

Eggs

WHY THEY'RE HEALTHY: They help burn fat, curb cravings, and build muscle, and they're loaded with nutrients.

HOW TO EAT THEM: However you like, just make sure you eat the yolks. The yellow stuff contains protein and vitamin B_{12}, which is necessary for fat breakdown.

BEST BET: Eggland's Best brand, packed with heart-healthy omega-3 fatty acids.

Berries

WHY THEY'RE HEALTHY: Berries protect your heart, improve your eyesight, enhance your memory, and prevent cravings.

HOW TO EAT THEM: Straight. Or you can add them to cereal, oatmeal, yogurt, or salads.

BEST BETS: raspberries, blueberries, strawberries

Tomatoes

WHY THEY'RE HEALTHY: They're loaded with vitamin C, lycopene, and beta-carotene.

HOW TO EAT THEM: Cooked tomatoes contain more cancer-fighting lycopene than raw tomatoes, so stir up some sauce or add them to your morning scrambled eggs.

BEST BET: If you're buying tomato sauce in a jar, avoid brands that are oversweetened with sugar. Sugar should be one of the last ingredients—not one of the first.

Why? Because if your weight is a battle between you and the natural mechanisms that drive your hunger, nature is going to win. You need to get nature on your side so it will encourage you to move in the right direction. Then it's not a fight, it's a cooperative enterprise. Let me describe some ways in which you're probably getting into trouble now, and how we'll deal with them:

If you're a slave to cravings . . . eat on a schedule. Have a meal or a snack every 3 hours, and balance their levels of fat, protein, and complex carbs (whole-grain crackers or whole fruits, for instance). This will keep your blood sugar steady; sugar crashes are the reason you have cravings in the first place. (Seriously, you'd have an easier time sleeping on a bed of nails than you would resisting a blood sugar crash.)

If you eat when you're stressed . . . give yourself a 20-minute stress break. Go for a walk, chew a piece of gum, or just stare at the wall and veg. Stress causes the release of the stress hormone cortisol, which is itself a powerful hunger inducer. The good news: It fades in your body after 20 minutes, when the calming hormone serotonin bounces back and sounds the all-clear. Knowing that this is the process will help you understand your hunger and tell it to just chill out.

If hunger visits you again and again during the day . . . have a glass of water. A region of the brain called the hypothalamus is the control center for both hunger and thirst, a design flaw that causes us endless confusion. And given how dehydrated the vast majority of us are, we're constantly misinterpreting what the hypothalamus is asking for. Give it a glass of water; your "hunger" will probably be satisfied. (By the way, if your pee is anything less than clear, you're probably dehydrated. Drink!)

If you're still desperate for food . . . have a stick of gum. The principle behind this goes back to that stress-and-food relationship I mentioned. In fact, Australian researchers who measured cortisol in the saliva of volunteers found that gum chewers had 16 percent less and responded better to stressful situations. Hey, it worked for the Doublemint twins.

If you're upset and at risk for a major binge . . . try dinner and a movie instead—and make it a comedy. Laughter cuts cortisol as well, and it releases the same feel-good endorphins that chowing on candy does. It even burns calories! One hour of laughing is equivalent to

30 minutes of working out, and much more fun. According to the American Film Institute, these are the 10 funniest movies of all time:

1. **Some Like It Hot**
2. **Tootsie**
3. **Dr. Strangelove**
4. **Annie Hall**
5. **Duck Soup**
6. **Blazing Saddles**
7. **M*A*S*H**
8. **It Happened One Night**
9. **The Graduate**
10. **Airplane!**

And somehow they missed *There's Something about Mary*, *Meet the Parents*, *Old School*, and *Caddyshack*!

Do I seriously consider watching a movie a weight-loss strategy?

I do and I don't. But there's an important principle represented by that movie list: Losing weight means tapping into all kinds of new ways of thinking, including knowing that on a night when you really want to down the whole carton of Ben and Jerry's, you can do something better for you instead.

In fact, "down" moods are a powerful reason that people overeat; the stress hormone cortisol literally tells your body it needs to store more fat. Three-quarters of people who lose weight and then gain some or all of it back eat unconsciously because of their emotions. When you consider the power of mind over body, a funny movie starts to make more sense than what's being said by 99 percent of the food police out there. Those weight-loss gurus are so focused on your belly that they ignore your mind.

And that's where *The Lean Belly Prescription* differs from all other weight-loss plans. Simply put, it's about letting more pleasure into your life: closer relationships, more energy to spend on having fun, more confidence in your body, more confidence in your future.

Your pursuit of all that has to be positive and life enhancing, just as it is when you see Jack Lemmon and Tony Curtis in full drag in *Some Like It Hot*. You laugh, and you burn calories—but the bigger point here is to laugh.

On some level, *The Lean Belly Prescription* is as much about less weight as it is about more joy.

10 SECOND SLIMDOWN

Motivation

A lot of people attempt to lose weight; only some of them succeed. What do the slimming success stories share? Smart strategies like these.

STEP OUTSIDE

University of Rochester scientists found that people who spent at least 20 minutes a day outdoors felt they had up to 20 percent more physical and mental energy than those who stayed inside. More research is needed to determine why, but the study authors ruled out the effects of exercise and socialization, which people do more of when they're outdoors. Can't finagle some fresh air? Open the blinds: Just eyeballing nature can recharge you.

DO IT FOR YOUR SEX LIFE

A study from Duke University showed that a 10 percent reduction in weight resulted in major improvements in all areas of the study participants' sex lives, including arousal, feelings of attractiveness, and enjoyment.

BE THE FAMILY THAT EATS TOGETHER

Food scientists at the University of Minnesota tracked the dining habits of a group of 12-year-olds. The ones who ate dinner with their families 5 days a week were likely to take in more calcium, fiber, and potassium in their late teens.

PROTECT YOUR BRAIN FROM SWEETS

Researchers at Tufts University found a link between carbs and mood. Men on low-sugar diets had lower levels of depression and anxiety than men who consumed all kinds of carbs. Happier people limited carbs to 40 percent of their diet.

RECOVER FROM TV

The negative health effects of watching television for 1 hour can be counterbalanced by 15 minutes of exercise. Makes you reconsider your romance with the remote, doesn't it?

TO CUT YOUR BMI, WORK OUT WITH YOUR SPOUSE

Researchers from the University of Alabama determined that overweight and obese people sacrifice 3 years from their life spans, compared with leaner people. Sedentary men are 50 percent more likely to work out three times a week if they do it with their partners, according to a study from Duke University.

CLEAN TO BE LEAN

A study done at Indiana University revealed that people with the cleanest houses also had the highest levels of physical activity. It's exercise with a purpose: Half an hour of mopping or vacuuming is about equal to a 15-minute jog.

PROVIDE A SOUNDTRACK

A study from the North American Association for the Study of Obesity found that women are much more likely to stick with an exercise program if they listen to music while they worked out.

PLAY WITH YOUR KIDS

Running around can be as beneficial as a formal workout, according to the *Journal of Sports Medicine and Physical Fitness*. Just 20 minutes of playing soccer or dodgeball raised adults' heartrates to 88 percent of their maximum and burned 160 calories; half an hour burned 240 calories—about the same as a moderate bike ride. The games were more than enough to produce benefits from physical activity, according to study coauthor Phillip Watts, Ph.D., of Northern Michigan University.

CHAPTER 3

Change Your Body, Change Your Life

The Lean Belly Prescription targets far more than just your waistline. Discover the benefits to your brain, your heart, and even your wallet!

~~~~~~~~~~~~~~~~~~~~~~~~~~~

S ome people might say that maintaining a lean belly is a mark of vanity. And they might be right. But when you consider all the benefits of *The Lean Belly Prescription*, well, a little more vanity might be a good thing!

You see, *The Lean Belly Prescription* isn't just about helping you cure your belly-fat emergency. It's also about making a huge impact on how you look, feel, and perform *physically, emotionally, professionally,* and *personally*. In fact, losing belly fat might just change your life in ways you can't imagine.

We humans are still part of the animal kingdom—a place where words are scarce, and where visual and physical cues still speak volumes. You can stand on the street corner all day long and declare that you're fit, healthy, and happy, but if your belly sags, if your posture is stooped, and if your face shows the evidence of too much stress and too little sleep, nobody's going to believe you. We're wired to give our five senses more credence than we give mere words.

But strip away that belly fat, and begin to enjoy all the physical and emotional benefits of a leaner, stronger, fitter you, and suddenly things change dramatically. Is getting back in shape "vain"? Maybe, but even Ben "A Penny Saved Is a Penny Earned" Franklin argued that a little more vanity wouldn't be such a bad thing. He wrote: "Most people dislike vanity, [but] I give it fair quarter wherever I meet with it, being persuaded that it is often productive of good to the possessor . . . and therefore, in many cases, it would not be altogether absurd if a man were to thank God for his vanity."

We are constantly judging each other as prospective mates, as rivals, as allies, and as friends by the physical signs each of us shows to the world. Vanity can help you show the best "you," the real "you," to everyone you meet. I've tried to impress upon you how urgent it is to lose belly fat, and how very bad things can get if you carry more than you should. But let's look at some of the other benefits of *The Lean Belly Prescription*—benefits that most doctors won't tell you about. But they should! For starters:

CHAPTER
3

LAWS OF
LEANNESS

"Vanity" is just another way of saying you're closely monitoring your health indicators.

Couples who exercise together stay together.

A LEAN BELLY MEANS MORE LOVE—AND MORE SEX!

It's not a huge leap of the imagination to figure that people who are lean and fit also have more vibrant sex lives. After all, we're not going to be seeing Kevin James on the cover of *People's* "Sexiest Men" issue any time soon. But the benefits of a lean belly go far beyond the expected. The spark of physical attraction is key, even if you're in a stable marriage to a wonderful spouse. Maybe *especially* if you're in a stable marriage with a wonderful spouse: Who wouldn't want more years to enjoy that special bond? I promise you will only become closer if you and your partner pair up to pursue *The Lean Belly Prescription*.

You'll feel more sexually alive. In a survey of 1,210 people of different weights and sizes conducted by Duke University Medical Center, obese people were 25 times more likely to report dissatisfaction with sex as normal-weight folks. And researchers at the University of Texas found that women who felt good about their bodies reported much greater levels of arousal and desire than those who felt bad about how they looked. But you don't need to sculpt yourself down to Aniston-esque dimensions to reap the benefits. Researchers at Duke say that *people report much greater enjoyment of sexual activity following a weight loss of just 10 percent!*

You'll improve your sexual response. Sexual function is all about capillaries—the small blood vessels that populate a man's penis and a woman's vagina. One of the negative effects of elevated blood sugar is that it damages blood vessels throughout the body, particularly in the feet, the eyes, and the genitals. Even if you aren't at risk for diabetes, the same arterial sludge that gunks up your heart arteries

Losing weight can cure back pain, joint pain, and heartburn, and improve sexual function.	Sleeping better helps you lose weight. Losing weight helps you sleep better.	Less weight means a longer life packed with more enjoyment.	Skinnier people are wealthier people. Smarter and happier, too.

will also affect blood flow below the belt—and not in a good way. But even people who engaged in moderate physical activity—the kind I outline for you in Chapter 6—were 65 percent less likely to report sexual problems. Indeed, subjects reported that kind of dramatic improvement after doing no more than taking a brisk 30-minute walk every other day.

You'll improve your relationship. It's a fairly simple concept, really. Couples who attempt great things together succeed together and bond through the experience. You'll improve your prospects for success with this plan by following it as a couple; and you'll improve your prospects for success as a couple by following this plan. That's the kind of win-win we can all enjoy.

A LEAN BELLY MEANS MORE SLEEP AND BETTER SLEEP!

Hey, as long as we're in bed already, let's linger there for a moment. Studies have repeatedly shown a link between fitness and sleep: If you engage in a little more physical activity—especially in the morning or at midday—you'll have better luck settling down for the evening and getting the sleep you need for memory storage, muscle repair, and sweet dreams. There are a number of reasons why.

You'll have less sleep-disrupting stress. In one study, Texas A&M University scientists found that the fittest people had lower levels of stress hormones in their bloodstreams than subjects who were least fit.

You'll fall asleep more naturally—when you want to! That's because exercise causes microscopic tears in your muscle fibers, and your body rushes special cells in to fix them. (Don't worry, that's a good thing—that's the process by which your body builds and maintains flab-burning muscle.) And just like the night crews that work on the busy interstate when there's little traffic, your muscle repair and strengthening processes take place largely while you sleep. That feeling of fatigue at night? It's your body telling you to take a load off so the repair crews can head in.

You'll snore less—meaning fewer jabs in the side. Having a big belly and a fatty neck can trigger chronic loud snoring and its partner, a sleep disorder called sleep apnea. People who have sleep

3 WAYS TO HAVE IT ALL

JUST FIVE 30-MINUTE CARDIO SESSIONS PER WEEK ARE ENOUGH
TO BOOST YOUR BRAINPOWER. SOUND DOABLE? AND SMART? IT IS.

1 *Wake up early.*

A 2005 study published in *Health Psychology* reported that it took new exercisers about 5 weeks to make their sessions a habit. And hitting the road at dawn doesn't mean you'll miss out on sleep. Researchers at Northwestern University found that people who started exercising in the morning slept better than they had before they began working out.

2 *Prioritize your life.*

Calculate the average time you spend daily doing everything from analyzing spreadsheets to watching TV. Once you've counted up those hours, you'll see that you can fit exercise in by deciding what's most important. Always give priority to activities that serve the greatest purpose—those involving work, family, and exercise. I have a rule: If I want to watch an hour of TV, I have to have exercised for 30 minutes that day. Earn your TV time! It's that simple.

3 *Call it multitasking.*

Exercise isn't work time lost; it's an opportunity to focus on job problems without distraction. If you do it with workmates, it's a brainstorming session. With the boss, it's face time. At home, exercising with your spouse or kids is quality time. It's all in how you define it.

apnea literally stop breathing for a few seconds or more, often hundreds of times a night. That causes them to wake up fatigued, even if they think they got 7 hours' sleep. And even if sleep apnea isn't a health issue, less snoring always means a more pleasant sleeping arrangement.

You'll replace daytime hunger with nighttime slumber. That's right: A lean belly means better sleep, and better sleep means a leaner belly. A study done at the University of Chicago put 12 men through a sleep-deprivation exercise. After 2 days of short sleep, their output of the hunger-inducing hormone ghrelin soared, while the hunger-reducing hormone leptin was suppressed. The result: Their cravings for high-carb, high-calorie foods increased by up to 45 percent. And a separate study done at Stanford University measured the body fat and hunger hormones of 1,000 people and found that those who slept less than 8 hours per night had lower leptin and higher ghrelin levels and more body fat. *The Lean Belly Prescription* will send you off in the right direction on the exercise–sleep–weight-loss charts.

A LEAN BELLY WILL MAKE YOU LOOK YOUNGER!

Of course, leaner people just naturally look younger—even more so in a world where almost everybody gets fat in middle age. But *The Lean Belly Prescription* does more than just that. You'll be stunned by the results.

You'll reverse aging at the cellular level. How? Meet the mighty mitochondria. You may never have heard of them, but they're the microscopic batteries that power your cells. When you exercise and eat right, you build more of them, so you're literally adding energy to your system. If you don't take care of your mitochondria, on the other hand, you'll discover the consequences: Aging has been described as a process of degrading the mitochondria—the equivalent of leaving your car's lights on overnight. But if you follow *The Lean Belly Prescription,* you'll keep your lights burning brightly. Here's how it works. The main function of mitochondria is to turn the nutrients

5 Rules of a Satisfied Belly

END YOUR BINGES FOR GOOD
WITH THE SECRETS OF A HAPPY STOMACH

It's happened to you before: You eat a meal and then you're hungry again, and scrambling for something else to wolf down. Stop the calorie cascade. You can prevent oversnacking and stop overeating with these five simple mind and body tricks for satisfaction.

1 *Just add water*

Your stomach is like a balloon. Fill it with anything—burgers, apples, rice—and you'll eventually feel full. A smarter way to fill your belly without stuffing it with calories is to take sips of water between bites of food. This will increase the bulk in your stomach, blowing up the balloon, and help you feel full more quickly without a calorie glut.

2 *Fill with fiber*

Fiber passes through your body undigested, slowing the absorption of nutrients and making you feel fuller longer, according to a 2008 review study by University of Minnesota researchers. Try adding high-fiber foods like whole-wheat pasta, raspberries, beans, and peas to your meals. See the list at LeanBellyRx.com to find out how much fiber some common foods have.

3 *Eat protein*

This nutrient has the ability to raise the level of peptides in your stomach. These little peptides relay messages telling your brain that your stomach is full. Aim for 20 to 40 grams of protein with every meal for the greatest benefit. At breakfast, two eggs, a slice of cheese, and a piece of whole-grain bread will do the trick. At lunch, ¾ cup of cottage cheese and a handful of nuts will work. To consume that amount at dinner, eat a 3-ounce filet mignon.

4 *Chew*

You heard me. Taking smaller bites and chewing your food longer may help you eat less at meals, according to a study published in the scientific journal *Physiology and Behavior*. If you slow down and enjoy your food, your brain has more time to register the eating process. In short: Don't take the term "slider" literally.

5 *Cut out distractions*

Eating while preoccupied impairs your brain's ability to watch your food intake, according to a 2009 review of studies. Turn off the TV, close the laptop, and stop playing games with your smartphone. Your stomach will thank you.

you eat into an energy molecule called adenosine triphosphate (ATP). Over time, the mitochondria run down, and produce enough waste products to do in their host cell. That is, unless you exercise and eat right. The more activity you do, the more energy your body requires, and the harder the mitochondria work. (Essentially the same way your car's battery wears out when it sits idle, but recharges itself as you drive.) So if you use 'em, you don't lose 'em. Meanwhile, your mitochondria are producing waste, in the form of the notorious "free radicals," which can damage cells, leading to aging. But by packing your day with more nutrition and fewer empty calories, you'll counteract the effects of these waste products. *The Lean Belly Prescription*, then, is like hiring the world's tiniest cosmetic surgeon to give your mitochondria a makeover, one cell at a time!

You'll look younger to those around you. Remember those capillaries that are feeding blood to your privates? They're also bringing blood to your skin and hair follicles to keep them supplied with energy to grow and repair tissues. Same with your eyes, teeth, and gums. So if you're overloading your system with added sugars or eating a lot of processed foods, you're sending your blood sugar on a roller-coaster ride that ultimately damages the health sign posts people most notice about you. In fact, a 2008 study of 186 pairs of identical female twins at Case Western Reserve University found that only a small part of facial aging had to do with genetics; most of what we call "aging" can be traced to lifestyle habits and environment. Researchers there found that the top two factors that accelerated aging were—no surprise here—sun damage and smoking. But a third, critical factor was weight.

A LEAN BELLY COULD MAKE YOU RICHER!

That sounds like a crazy claim, doesn't it? Consider what top researchers are saying about the power of a flat tummy.

Your family income might increase. The Centers for Disease Control and Prevention asked people across the economic spectrum about their exercise habits. Among the people with the lowest family incomes—$35,000 or less—about 24 percent included regular

3 Mood-Lifting Workouts

IT'S SIMPLE: THE MORE ACTIVE YOU ARE,
THE HAPPIER YOU'LL BE

1
Trigger nature's antidepressants.

Exercise pumps up not only the mood-regulating neurotransmitter serotonin, but also levels of dopamine and norepinephrine, two other natural happiness helpers. Plus, physical activity makes it easier for tryptophan (a building block of serotonin) to enter the brain, says Daniel Amen, M.D., an assistant professor of psychiatry at the University of California, Irvine.

THE WORKOUT
You don't need an intense gym session—walking or jogging for 15 minutes at lunchtime will do the trick.

2
Heat up so you can chill out.

Exercise triggers the white blood cells to release pyrogens, peptides that increase the body's temperature by 1° to 2°F. The result: a soothing, full-body heat wave. "Working out has a calming effect very similar to that of spending time in a sauna or a hot shower, and all three can help relieve anxiety and depression," says Larry Leith, Ph.D., author of *Exercising Your Way to Better Mental Health.*

THE WORKOUT
Exercise your large muscle groups by cycling, swimming, or lifting weights for at least 20 minutes. "That's how long it takes to achieve the temperature change," Leith says.

3
Interrupt negative thoughts.

Working out stops self-destructive mind games; if your workday is a source of your angst, interrupting the flow could be a real help. "Exercise gives a sense of self-mastery, and that's a powerful coping mechanism," says Keith Johnsgard, Ph.D., author of *Conquering Depression and Anxiety through Exercise.*

THE WORKOUT
Choose a sport you loved playing as a kid and get back in the game. "If you go back to an activity that made you feel good, it's likely that those neural pathways will be stimulated again," says William Pollack, Ph.D., a professor of psychiatry at Harvard Medical School and a *Men's Health* advisor.

physical exercise in their weekly plans. Among families earning $100,000 or more, 45 percent did. Now, it's fair to ask whether lower-income families were time-poor, as well, and thus couldn't find a moment to schedule exercise. But you can't help noting that the best fitness habits seem to run together with high earnings.

Your company will see you as more promotable. An economics professor at the University of Texas at Austin performed a series of studies he called "Beauty and the Labor Market," detailing the effects of vanity (that word again!) in the business world. He discovered that people with above-average looks tended to be paid about 5 percent more than plain-looking people, and that people who had below-average looks could be penalized by up to 9 percent. When you do the math, you find that *going from overweight to having a lean belly could result in as much as a 15.4 percent wage increase.* What's more, the employers are getting their money's worth. Dutch researchers found that advertising agencies with the best-looking employees brought in the most revenue. Even though they had to pay the good-looking people more, their extra revenues more than made up for the disparity in wages. Obviously we're not saying *The Lean Belly Prescription* will make you look like Angelina Jolie or Brad Pitt. But don't we all look and feel more confident when we're not carrying excess cargo? Another study showed that the tasks a non-exerciser would need 9.5 hours to accomplish would be handled by an exerciser in 8 hours. Given that productivity boost, a pay boost is only reasonable. (Have your boss call me; I'll explain it all to him.)

A LEAN BELLY
WILL MAKE YOU SMARTER!

If you're already younger, leaner, richer, and sexier, not to mention better rested, wouldn't becoming smarter just be overkill? Maybe, but the type of nutrition and exercise advice in *The Lean Belly Prescription* has been shown to subtly rewire brain circuitry known as P3, which speeds the transmission of messages and improves memory and focus. Indeed, a smaller belly seems to lead naturally to a bigger brain, for many reasons.

Exercising your body helps you make smart choices. A famous

THE THINKING MAN'S

(and Woman's)

EXERCISE PLAN

The research is clear: Thirty minutes of exercise makes you smarter—immediately. But what about the effects of 20 minutes, or even 10? I say any activity is better than none and gives you the means to build up to the amount the scientists tested. Here's all you need to know to achieve the brain-sharpening effects you're after.

Duration

Keep moving for 30 minutes. Any cardio exercise will do—running, cycling, swimming, rowing. In fact, it's best to diversify, especially if you're a beginner, to avoid overuse injuries.

Frequency

Do your cardio anytime you want a mental boost. For the long haul, doing as few as three sessions a week has been shown to improve the mental performance of older adults, says Charles Hillman, Ph.D., associate professor of kinesiology and public health at the University of Illinois. So consider that your minimum.

Intensity

Even walking appears to have brain benefits, but you need to pick up the pace to ensure that you replicate the results of Hillman's research. His subjects exercised at "somewhat hard" or "hard" levels for the duration of their sessions. It's a "perceived exertion" scale, so you can't mess up: Just use your own judgment.

experiment at Purdue University in 1986 followed 30 women who were put on an exercise program. As their fitness levels rose by 17 percent, their measured success in sound decision making and information processing rose by between 12 and 68 percent. That early study launched a whole new field of inquiry in exercise science and led to a 2003 study at the University of Illinois at Urbana-Champaign. College students worked out for 30 minutes on two separate occasions, taking tests before and after their sweat sessions. The results: After exercise, the test subjects showed better decision making, improved memory, and longer attention spans.

The researchers then repeated the test, but recruited people of different ages as the test subjects. The older adults who regularly exercised had faster reaction times and better accuracy on tests than the sedentary adults.

People who exercise are sharper at work. Researchers at Leeds Metropolitan University in England had workers answer questionnaires about their job performance on days when they didn't exercise and on days when they did. They rated their ability to work continuously and how well they did with their to-do lists. The results: The workers performed 15 percent better on both time and output demands on days when they worked out. These same workers also reported feeling less stressed and enjoying their jobs more. These benefits will serve you well when your boss asks you for a snap analysis, but what about the longer-term effects?

A lean belly will protect your brain as you age. There has been a rash of recent studies that link belly fat in middle age to dementia—including Alzheimer's disease—3 decades later. One study, released in 2007, tracked 6,000 people under the care of Kaiser Permanente doctors. Subjects' waists were measured in the late 1960s and early '70s, and then their mental diagnoses were tracked 30 years later. The finding: *People who stored fat in their bellies were more than three times as likely to suffer from dementia later on in life.*

The people with less belly fat—like you, say, 4 weeks from now—cut their risk of insulin imbalances destroying the brain's ability to process memories, which one researcher has called "type 3 diabetes." Incredibly, the more belly fat you can lose today, the more likely you'll remain focused, aware, and vital well into your later years.

And Alzheimer's isn't the only brain-related malady that has been linked to belly fat. It's also an indicator for depression, anxiety, and stroke. If you want to keep your mind sharp, you'll want to make sure your belly is lean.

A LEAN BELLY
WILL MAKE YOU HAPPIER!

Okay, really now: You're younger, leaner, richer, sexier, *and* smarter. What's not to be happy about? But in fact, research shows that following *The Lean Belly Prescription* will make you happier in addition to all those things. Want proof?

You'll boost your levels of feel-good brain chemicals. Researchers at Duke University determined that moderate-intensity cardio, performed three times a week, was as effective as the antidepressant sertraline (Zoloft) for treating depression. One possible explanation: Exercise increases the amounts of several feel-good neurotransmitters in your blood, so it gives your mood a boost. It also ups the level of communication between different regions of your brain, allowing you to come up with innovative solutions to problems you face. For instance, that belly fat problem you *used* to have, right?

You'll eat scientifically proven "happy foods." It sounds too good to be true, but a study in the journal *Psychotherapy and Psychosomatics* shows that low levels of folate—a nutrient found in abundance in nuts, beans, and leafy greens (and in *The Lean Belly Prescription*)—are typically found in people with depression. Another study found that adding folate-rich foods to your diet reduces fatigue, improves energy levels, and helps battle the blues.

There's a whole new world of wellness out there for you, once you commit to *The Lean Belly Prescription*. I can't promise you a six-pack in 6 weeks, or that you'll instantly be able to squeeze back into jeans you last wore in high school. But if you commit to PICK 3 TO LEAN—if you simply choose the options that appeal to you, and give them a spin, and mix in just one of the incredibly easy exercise options in Chapter 6—then all of the benefits of *The Lean Belly Prescription* can be yours!

10 SECOND SLIMDOWN

Body Benefits!

Weight loss isn't just about going down a few notches on your belt. It's about improving your life in dozens of significant ways. If you've got 10 seconds, you're on your way.

MOVE IT

French scientists have found that the type of exercise you do doesn't matter, as long as you're moving. Accumulate a total of 4 hours over the course of 3 to 4 days, and you'll join the ranks of people with the leanest midsections.

BE NOTICED AT WORK

When dining out with co-workers, don't follow the overeating crowd—it could benefit your career. "If your boss and colleagues see you eating healthfully, you're going to look like an outcome-driven leader," says behavioral therapist Robinson Welch, Ph.D. "It sends a message that you want to be successful. That you'll take care of business the same way you take care of yourself—effectively."

CUSHION YOUR WALLET

Slashing just 100 calories a day—about 18 Cheez-Its' worth—from your diet will save you an average of $175.20 a year.

HAVE MORE FRIENDS

Fit people are more fun to be around. Check this out: One study looked at kids who played outdoors and kids who spent their time indoors. The ones who went outside to play were more popular with other kids. And, oddly, their parents were more popular, too!

SAVE YOUR SEX DRIVE

Lose your gut to save your passion. According to a landmark 2007 study in the *Journal of Clinical Endocrinology and Metabolism,* men with a 5-point increase in body mass index—about 30 extra pounds—had testosterone levels comparable to men who were a full decade older.

SHINE YOUR SMILE

Drinking milk may help preserve the enamel on your teeth, according to a study from the University of Iowa. Add that to dairy's rep as a weight buster, and you'll be looking better on two fronts.

PAIR UP FOR BETTER RESULTS

Healthy eaters subconsciously influence their spouses to lose weight, say University of Connecticut researchers. "Couples support each other by working together," says study author Amy Gorin, Ph.D.

SNACK FIRST!

Going to a party? Have a big snack beforehand. It'll help you dodge the high-calorie hazards of the buffet line.

SKYROCKET SEXUAL SATISFACTION

A survey of 1,210 people of different weights and sizes conducted by researchers at Duke University Medical Center showed that obese people were 25 times as likely to report dissatisfaction with sex as normal weight people. The magic elixir: the Duke study, and others, show that a simple 10 percent loss of body weight skyrockets sex satisfaction levels.

WALK AROUND THE BLOCK, BE BETTER IN BED

A study of 178 healthy men at the Durham VA Medical Center in North Carolina showed that walking for 30 minutes a day, 4 days a week, boosted scores on a sex survey. And the more exercise respondents did, the more they enjoyed sex.

CHAPTER 4

Your
PICK 3
TO LEAN
Prescription

Lose belly fat fast, without dieting!
Here's the easiest, most delicious
eating plan you'll ever find!

~~~~~~

"**O**kay, fine, Dr. Travis. But when do we eat?" I understand why you might be getting hungry. After all, this is an eating plan that lets you enjoy all your favorite foods while getting leaner, sexier, richer, smarter, and happier—and living longer. Pass the food already!

I gave you an appetizer portion of PICK 3 TO LEAN in the introduction. And a little further along in this chapter, I'll lay out that smorgasbord in more detail. But first, I'd like to address a pressing question that more and more patients seem to ask me:

"How did we all get so darn fat?"

Two-thirds of American adults are either overweight or obese. Two out of three. Think about that. How did this happen?

It started a few decades back, with a statement that sounds pretty familiar: *Eat less fat.*

It seems to make sense, right? If you eat fat, you get fat; if you avoid fat, well, you'll stay slim forever.

Let me cut through the nutritional clutter and get straight to the point: Nothing has had a more damaging effect on our national waistline than those three little words.

It may feel like we've been living in the United States of Obesity forever, but as recently as the mid-1980s, it wasn't nearly as prevalent as it is now. According to Centers for Disease Control and Prevention statistics, not one state had an obesity rate of higher than 15 percent back in those lean times. But in 2007, 49 states admitted that 20 percent (or more) of their citizens were obese. Not just overweight, but obese—meaning that their health was at risk from their weight. Given what we know about belly fat and chronic disease, it's no wonder that health-care costs are skyrocketing.

It all came from the *big fat mistake*—there, I said it—that fat makes you fat. The reality: It's the combination of excessive eating, simple carbs, and unhealthy fats (fried foods, trans fats) that piled up in the national diet, creating a bellyquake of historic proportions.

Here's how it happened. In the 1950s, theories were circulating around how cholesterol—fat molecules in the blood—played a role in

CHAPTER
4

LAWS OF
LEANNESS

| Fat (in moderation!) doesn't make you fat. It fills your belly and keeps you satisfied. | Americans drink an average of 450 calories a day. Drop sugary drinks, and you'll drop pounds. |

heart disease. "Aha!" the nutritionists of the day cried. "There's choles-terol in fatty foods! Ergo: Fatty foods cause heart disease. If you care about your heart, stop eating them immediately!"

So we did.

People quickly came to equate "low fat" with "healthy," and the food manufacturers responded by inventing new types of foods, foods that looked a lot like what we used to eat—and tasted kinda like what we used to eat—but whose labels could now sport words like "no fat," "low fat," and "low cholesterol." And everyone assumed they were guideposts to better health.

The problem: The scientists were wrong about fat.

IT'S TIME TO START ENJOYING FOOD AGAIN!

We now know that many types of fat are, in fact, among the best things you can eat for heart health. Your body also digests fats very slowly, so your feeling of fullness sticks with you after you eat them. In other words, fat helps you control your appetite. Reduce fat, and you often wind up ingesting more calories. You still have to watch the amounts and types of fat you eat, but if you use it the right way it can be a tool for good health *and* a lean waistline.

And we now know that there's a big difference between the cholesterol you eat and the cholesterol in your blood. So the "no cholesterol" label on that tub of margarine is true enough, but it won't have any positive impact on your health. We used to be impressed by people who ordered egg-white omelettes; now they're

The fewer ingredients your food contains, the fewer pounds you'll gain.	You can still enjoy fatty foods— eggs, steak, butter, even bacon.	Avoid diets; instead, alter your lifestyle to lose weight for a lifetime.	The low-fat craze scared us straight into the arms of the real monster: sugar.

just demonstrating their ignorance every time they order one. (The yolk has tons of useful nutrients, is low in calories, and looks like a sunrise over farm country.)

So one thing you'll discover as you make your PICK 3 TO LEAN choices is that steak, eggs, and even butter are on your list of acceptable food options. You can even have a couple of strips of bacon with your eggs, if you like. It will curb your appetite much more in the long run than a bagel which high-sugar jelly. A little more fat in your diet now will help you avoid a lot of useless calories later.

What kind of useless calories? Why, simple carbs, of course. Because when the big fat mistake happened, we replaced fatty foods—natural appetite suppressants—with high-carbohydrate foods, which are to appetite what gasoline is to fire. We were taking in much more energy than we could possibly use so we stored it in the form of body fat. So scientists had sold us on the idea that "fat makes you fat," but the truth was actually the opposite: Avoiding fat made us fat. How's that for a (big) surprise ending?

THE FOOD MISTAKE THAT'S MADE US FAT

Let's look at what happens when you eat refined carbohydrates, which are essentially simple chains of molecules. These carbs are easy energy for the human body, but hard to find in nature—we developed our sweet tooth so we'd seek out berries and other high-nutrient fruits, which were among the only real sources of these sugars in the natural world. So our bodies are built to seek them out constantly, and to digest them rapidly.

As soon as they hit your mouth, your saliva starts breaking them down and your brain throws a party: *Sweet*, it says, *keep on eating!* When you eat a slice of white bread, your digestive tract reacts as if it's 4 tablespoons of sugar: It instantly breaks down those simple carbs into glucose, a blood sugar that can be used to fuel all the activities you pursue, from mere breathing to running a marathon. But if you fail to show up at the race, what happens to all that stored energy? Your body uses the hormone insulin to shepherd excess glucose into fat cells.

Early on in your life, your body is very efficient at doing this. Insulin flows, and it mops up all the extra glucose in your bloodstream and packs it into your muscle, fat, brain, and other organs' cells. But as we become older and less active, our bodies become less efficient with glucose. A lifetime of too much soda and sitting on the couch will cause insulin to preferentially guide glucose into your fat cells. (Your muscles clearly don't need it!) So after each high-calorie meal, sure enough, your body's 50 billion fat cells get their next load of energy. And each fat cell gets even fatter.

That, multiplied by 160 million people, is what was happening in our country during the '80s, '90s, and the early part of this century.

Now let's turn ourselves to a healthier process, the one that happens when you broaden your diet to include more fat, fiber, protein, and whole grains. I'm talking about milk and cheese here, and luscious Greek yogurt. I'm talking about a steak sizzling on the grill, or a salmon fillet encrusted with pepper and herbs. What do these foods all have in common? Two things: They all contain fat. And they all can be really good for you.

A balanced meal mixes carbs with fat, fiber, and protein, which take longer to process. Your digestive process has to work hard to break down all the complex molecular structures, so the process is relatively slow. Energy is slowly released into your bloodstream, so the insulin has more time to shuttle energy to where it can be used, instead of just stashing it in your fat cells. Your blood sugar level remains constant rather than swooping and crashing, and there's time for your gut to signal your brain that it has enough energy, you can stop eating now.

So there's no struggle to "control" your appetite. There's no sacrifice. You just eat good, nutritious, even fatty foods, and then your body lets you know when it's satisfied. How great is that?

That doesn't sound like a diet to me. It sounds like satisfaction.

YES, FINALLY, NOW WE GET TO EAT!

You'll find eight proven food strategies in this chapter, each of which can help you lose at least 2—and overall as much as 15—pounds in the next 4 weeks. And you'll notice that not one of them requires you to go into starvation mode, to count calories, or to eat low-fat, low-carb, low-anything. Each is a simple, easy-to-follow tweak to your current eating habits, but each can make a dramatic change in the way you look and feel.

And here's the part I love: You don't have to do all eight. Instead, I'm simply asking you to start with any three items off the menu. And you'll base your choices not on what you're willing to give up, but on what you love to eat. Enjoy carbs? You'll eat better, healthier carbs, and still lose up to 2 pounds a week. Like to drink soda? I can give you a simple switch that will strip away up to 4 pounds in just the next month. Big fan of breakfast? Prepare to lose nearly a pound every single week! But if you're not a fan of carbs, soda or breakfast, don't worry—there are five more options to choose from.

How will you enjoy all this food without turning into a walrus? Flip to the box on page 41, called "Five Rules of a Satisfied Belly." Using techniques like that, you're going to crowd out the foods and behaviors that are now making you fat with better options I'll present in these pages. Instead of mindlessly filling your mouth while you watch TV, you'll concentrate more on every bite, enjoy them more, and take fewer of them quite naturally. Instead of wolfing down the whole box of carbs (cookies), you'll snack on equally delicious foods that will satisfy your hunger, not intensify it. You're going to swap the sweet sodas that are adding 450 calories a day to your diet for a zero-calorie beverage your body craves. These and other choices—PICK 3!—will lead to leanness just as surely as your old habits led to the opposite.

If you let your body operate the way nature designed it, it will cure your belly fat once and for all.

Now, a question: Why three food changes? Wouldn't it be simpler to start with just one? Actually, three's the scientifically proven charm.

In a Baylor College of Medicine study, one group of adults took on three simultaneous health goals, while a second group attempted a single goal. Eighteen months later, those who had embraced multiple healthy changes were 20 percent more likely to have stuck with them. The reason: Three changes are mutually reinforcing—they're a lifestyle, not just a lame resolution—so that committing to each individually helps you stick with all of them.

Once you see the change PICK 3 can make, why not try more? In fact, the more you choose, the more you lose.

But three is all you need to start seeing a dramatic difference: It's my PICK 3 TO LEAN plan—a shortcut to the fit, trim body you've always wanted! So here's your menu; eat what you love, and love how you look.

PICK 3 TO LEAN!

"I love cheese and yogurt!"

Who doesn't? And more and more evidence suggests that eating at least three (that number again) servings of calcium-rich dairy a day can strip fat away like magic. Harvard Medical School researchers found that people who ate three servings of dairy foods daily (containing 1,200 mg of calcium) were 60 percent less likely to be overweight than people who consumed less. And a study in *Molecular Systems Biology* found that yogurt-based bacteria can also reduce the amount of fat the body can absorb during digestion. If you love cheese and yogurt, eat at least three servings per day—have a glass of milk with breakfast, snack on cheese at lunchtime, or eat Greek yogurt for an afternoon snack. Or just stick with the yogurt: A University of Tennessee study found that people who added three servings of yogurt a day to their diets lost 81 percent more belly fat over 12 weeks than those who didn't eat yogurt! Just beware of the ones with tons of added sugar!

A GREAT OPTION: 1 cup of yogurt, 1 cup of milk, and 1½ ounces of real cheese every day

YOU COULD LOSE: 3 pounds in 4 weeks!

"I love pasta and rice!"

Then go for it. Just learn to love the whole-grain versions of your favorite foods, and nowadays, there are plenty available. I personally love carbs, but I've replaced white bread with whole wheat, and white rice with brown. I scan labels to screen out unnecessary sugars and artifical sweeteners. The reward: Penn State researchers say people who ate whole grains lost twice the belly fat of people who ate refined carbs! If you love carbs, switch all your refined carbs—white bread, white rice, regular pasta, and refined-flour products like crackers and cookies—to whole-grain versions. The study authors credit the extra fiber and antioxidants in whole grains, which help control insulin (the hormone that tells your body to store belly fat). And while you're at it, adjust the ratios of toppings to carbs in the dishes you love. In Italy, noodles are a side dish, not the main course. If you serve sauces thick with lean meat or vegetables, you'll gain protein, nutrients, and fiber, and still eat the pasta you love.

A GREAT OPTION: Replace your refined carbs with whole-wheat and whole-grain varieties, and make sure you're combining them with plenty of lean meats, vegetables, and healthy fats.

YOU COULD LOSE: 8 pounds in 4 weeks!

"I love soda!"

Then keep on drinking; it's an important way to fill your belly. But we're going to find new ways for you to get that soda buzz. Why make any change at all? A study in the *American Journal of Clinical Nutrition* found that we're consuming about 450 calories a day from sweetened beverages, more than twice what we were consuming 30 years ago. Sodas and other sugary beverages like sweet teas, energy drinks, and sports drinks now account for more than 20 percent of the calories we take in every day. So it's the first place you should look to cut; it may be the easiest. And another study, from Johns Hopkins University, found that cutting liquid calories had a greater impact on weight loss than cutting food calories. That's why, potentially, this could be the most effective of any of these tips in helping you lose weight—especially if you're in the throes of a soda addiction (the caffeine, sweetness, and craving for liquids can do that to you). So if you love soda, I want you to commit to a drinking program. One 8-ounce glass of water when you first wake up, another mid-morning, another before lunch, another mid-afternoon, another before dinner, and one at around 8 p.m. Put ice in that water, and you'll burn nearly 500 calories a week! (It's because your body has to expend calories in order to heat the ice water up to body temperature.) Plus, you'll find your belly fuller, your thirst less intense, and the soda monkey off your back while adding zero calories to your diet. For a ton of terrific options to replace sweet drinks for more wholesome ones, flip to page 64, and bottoms up! I drink (lemon sparkling water) to your success!

A GREAT OPTION: Any time you have an urge for soda or a sugary beverage, swap in a drink from page 64. Add my ice-water program and you'll kick the habit in 4 weeks!

YOU COULD LOSE: 4 pounds in 4 weeks!

"I love to graze!"

Then munch on fruits and vegetables all day long. A study in the *British Journal of Nutrition* found that dieters who ate the most folate—found in leafy greens like spinach and romaine—lost 8.5 times more weight than those who ate the least. And a UCLA study found that the average person of normal weight consumed at least two servings of fruit a day, while the average overweight person consumed only one. If you love munching on a variety of foods, eat at least two pieces of fruit every day and at least three servings of vegetables, focusing on leafy greens like spinach, broccoli and brussels sprouts. While you're at it, add a cup of beans to your regimen. A study in the *Journal of the American College of Nutrition* found that people who eat ¾ cup of beans each day have smaller waists and lower blood pressure than those who eat other proteins. A cup of cooked black, kidney, lima, or garbanzo beans contains more than 10 grams of hunger-stomping fiber. Want to rev up your body's natural fat burners at the same time? Add hot sauce. The heat-producing ingredient—capsaicin—may improve your liver's ability to clear insulin (the fat-storage hormone) from your bloodstream after a meal. Remember: Beans and greens mean lean!

A GREAT OPTION: A piece of whole fruit with breakfast, a leafy green salad with extra veggies for lunch, a serving of beans with dinner, and a serving of berries as a dessert or snack.

YOU COULD LOSE: 6 pounds in 4 weeks!

"I love breakfast!"

So do a lot of skinny people, and you can join them if you eat eggs, ham, bacon, dairy, or other forms of protein first thing. A Purdue study shows that eating more protein for breakfast helps people avoid overeating for the rest of the day. Another study in the *International Journal of Obesity* showed that eating two eggs instead of a bagel every morning allowed dieters to lose 65 percent more weight over 8 weeks. And eating breakfast regularly cuts your risk of obesity by 78 percent! If you love breakfast, make sure you eat it regularly and include both protein (milk, eggs, yogurt, quinoa), whole grains (cereal, steel-cut oats, whole-wheat toast, quinoa again), and whole fruit or berries (not fruit juice—even OJ has tons of concentrated sugar and no fiber, so whole fruit is much healthier). For more ideas on how to wake up and lose weight, flip to page 95, and read "What About Breakfast?"

A GREAT OPTION: Any of the Wake-Up Weight-Loss All-Stars on page 95. Choose the options you like!

YOU COULD LOSE: 4 pounds in 4 weeks!

"I love to snack!"

Good! If you snack in a smart way, you'll build more healthy foods into your diet, keep your belly full, and avoid the binge eating that leads to huge calorie payloads. So if you love snacking, make a snack using three food groups, and make sure at least one of them is protein. Examples: cheese (dairy/protein) + pear (fruits/vegetables) + whole-grain crackers (complex carbs). Or a banana (fruit) + peanut butter (legumes/protein) + a glass of milk (dairy/protein). Or turkey (protein) + tomato (vegetable) on a whole-wheat tortilla (complex carbs). Eating a three-part snack like this about two hours before mealtime will dramatically decrease the amount you eat later on. And by the way, plenty of your favorite foods will work quite well at snack time. A study presented at the Experimental Biology conference in 2009 showed that people who ate 1 cup of microwave popcorn (whole grain!) 30 minutes before lunch consumed 105 fewer calories at the meal than people who snacked on a cup of potato chips. Moreover, the popcorn had 15 calories; the chips had 150. In another study, people who consumed dark chocolate, ate 15 percent fewer calories in their next meal. Plus, they showed less interest in fatty, salty and sugary foods. Just make sure it's a specialty dark chocolate, with at least 65 percent cacao content. The goal here: Have a reasonably sized snack (2 tablespoons peanut butter, a handful of celery sticks, 8-ounce glass of milk) to undercut your appetite, and keep you from a big indescretion at the vending machine, or at dinner. Check out other "Trim Trio" options on page 127. Use good foods to manage hunger and they'll manage your waist size and health risks, too!

A GREAT OPTION: Two 200-calorie snacks every day—one mid-morning, the other midafternoon. Combine protein (nuts, yogurt, cheese) with whole grain (crackers, black bean chips, pita), and produce (fruit, celery, carrots).

YOU COULD LOSE: 7 pounds in four weeks!

"I love milk shakes!"

Then make them a cornerstone of your diet—with a few healthy, delicious modifications. In a study in the *European Journal of Nutrition*, those who drank a high-protein smoothie for breakfast consumed the fewest calories at lunchtime. As we learned above, adding three servings of yogurt to your daily diet can cause you to lose 81 percent more belly fat over 12 weeks—so make it the main ingredient in your smoothie. If you love milk shakes, have a yogurt/fruit/whey powder-based smoothie for breakfast and another in place of dessert or as a snack. You can find a ton of great recipes at LeanBellyRx.com.

A GREAT OPTION: Two smoothies per day for a meal replacement and snack. Blend 1½ cup fruit or berries with 1 cup yogurt or milk and 1 tablespoon each of peanut butter and protein powder. (Add ½ cup of water if it's too thick for your liking.)

YOU COULD LOSE: 4 pounds in 4 weeks!

"I love fatty foods!"

Then use it as one of your great allies in the fight against belly fat. Researchers at Brigham and Women's Hospital in Boston put 101 overweight people on either a low-fat diet or a moderate-fat diet and followed them for 18 months. Both groups lost weight, but only the moderate-fat group lost an average of 9 pounds per person and kept it off after a year. Healthy fats can lower your heart-disease risk by a third, chop your Alzheimer's risk by two-thirds, and help you slim down, partly because they take a long time to digest, and keep your belly fuller, longer. A possible prime source of healthy fat in our diets: beef! New studies show that conjugated linoleic acid (CLA) in beef fat helps reduce obesity risk and heart disease risk. A Swedish study showed that those who ate the most CLA after 4 weeks had the smallest bellies. Grass-fed beef has much higher concentrations of CLA. This isn't an invitation to stuff down hot dogs on refined-flour rolls, or to attempt the burget diet. If you love beef, choose low-fat cuts like sirloin, and opt for grass-fed varieties whenever possible. Protein means lean, too!

You're also free to snack every day on peanuts, peanut butter (the no-sugar-added kind), and other kinds of nuts. Don't be afraid to add shaved almonds or walnuts to your salad. Cook with olive oil, and if you like, go ahead and top vegetables with a pat of butter (it'll actually help you absorb nutrients better). It's okay to stir some whole cream into your coffee. Snack on string cheese or avocado slices. And enjoy whole-fat yogurts and cheeses. Now, I'm not giving you a free pass to eat the whole pot roast, or the wheel of cheese—these are calorie-dense foods, so you need to limit portions. Surround them with vegetables, fruits, and whole grains to fill your belly with other healthy nutrients. You'll notice how I did not recommend fried foods or any other fatty processed products like salad dressing. There's a reason for that. (If your fats come from real, not overly processed foods, and if you enjoy them in moderation and allow them to satisfy your appetite, then fat will not make you "fat.") In fact, if you include the right kinds and amounts of fat in your diet you'll actually keep it from gathering around your belly. (We'll talk more about healthy fats later.)

A GREAT OPTION: Have eggs at breakfast, a handful of nuts at 10 a.m., a salad with avocado at lunch, cheese rolled up in a slice of ham for a snack, and a reasonably sized steak (6 ounces or less) or salmon filet at dinner.

YOU COULD LOSE: 4 pounds in 4 weeks!

So there you are—the PICK 3 TO LEAN plan in a nutshell. (And if you've been reading carefully, you now know that nutshells nearly always contain good things.) Pick your three food approaches, enjoy them in moderation, and your life will change dramatically. After making three changes, I believe you'll want to try others. There's plenty of overlap and, as I've said, if you choose more, you lose more.

It's that simple, and it's that profound.

What's more, it's better than any prescription pill you've ever swallowed, because it's free, it's guaranteed effective, and the only side effects are positive ones—closer relationships, more and better sex, a lean look, and perhaps a surprised nod from your doctor the next time you go in for a routine physical.

But I won't be surprised at the change. I prescribed it, after all.

Cut the Carb Confusion

HOW TO MAKE A "COMPLEX" PROBLEM "SIMPLE"

You've probably heard a thousand times that there are two types of carbohydrates: simple and complex. But if you're like most people, you're probably finding this distinction somewhat complex, and not at all simple to understand. And what does "refined" mean, anyway? Here's an easy way to think about it:

Complex carbs

are strings of complex sugar molecules that take your body time to digest. They're found in whole foods like oats, nuts, whole-grain bread, corn on the cob, and the like. Whenever you see the words "whole grain," you know you're eating complex carbs, and you're doing your body a favor. Because it takes your body time to break down complex carbs, you get a slow, steady flow of energy, just like when you keep your foot on the accelerator at a steady 55 mph. You'll also get plenty of healthy vitamins, minerals, and fiber, too.

Simple carbs

are sugars that are found naturally in fruits, vegetables, and even dairy products. Eat them in those forms, and they come with a payload of fiber, fat, protein, or nutrients, which slow digestion and limit how much you'll eat or drink. That's not true of another simple carb: sugar (and its close cousin fructose). In candy, soda, and even fruit juice, these simple carbs rocket through your system and are likely to be stored as fat. Just like . . .

Refined carbs

When food manufacturers take complex carbs (whole wheat, for instance) and strip out all the fiber and many of the nutrients, they turn them into refined carbs. Think white bread. Another example: high-fructose corn syrup, a kind of Franken-sweetener that should scare you off from products that contain it. Refined carbs, along with pure sugar, are lean-belly enemies number one and two. Beware!

KICK YOUR SODA HABIT

AND DROP A POUND A WEEK!

Cutting down on soda calories is the fastest, easiest way to lose weight and improve your health. Emerging research suggests that even sugary-tasting "diet" drinks may lead to a higher risk for weight gain. Break the habit and swap in drinks that taste great, but won't inflate.

Flavored seltzer water

You'll find a whole shelf of them in the beverage aisle, flavored with everything from lemon and lime to vanilla, raspberry, and grapefruit. A store brand will cost about 70 cents for 32 ounces, and the flavoring and fizz—with zero calories—go a long way toward making them ideal soda substitutes. Just make sure you pick the ones without sugar, high fructose corn syrup, and artificial sweeteners— and start pushing those unwanted, unnecessary calories out of your life.

Homemade low-calorie soda

Even some bottled 100% juices have as many carbohydrates as soda. Those carbs come from

natural sugars instead of the artificial sugars in soda, but you still have to be careful about drinking extra calories. The solution: Fill a glass a third of the way with juice, and then fill the rest with seltzer. You'll defuse the potential sugar bomb, cut calories, and stretch your dollar.

TRY

- 100% cranberry juice **+** seltzer **=** a less bitter, more mellow cranberry concoction

- Apple cider **+** seltzer **=** sparkling apple cider

- Orange juice **+** seltzer **=** virgin mimosa

- Seltzer **+** a squirt of bottled lemon or lime juice **=** citrus "soda"

- Pineapple juice **+** a dash of pomegranate juice **+** seltzer **=** faux tropical cocktail

Real iced tea

Sugar-loaded sweet teas packed with corn syrup have turned tea into an enemy. Real iced tea, the unsweetened variety brewed without additives, contains diseasefighting antioxidant power and is a naturally no-calorie, flavorful beverage. Too bland? Gussy up your tea with tastebud pleasers and you'll get rid of that giant jug of sugar water sitting in your fridge.

TRY

- Jasmine tea **+** a lemon wedge **=** one calming cup

HEALTH BONUS: The scent of jasmine may have the power to calm your nerves, according to German researchers. Plus, lemon may boost your mood, according to a separate study. Stress is a major weight booster, so a calming drink could have double the benefits.

Black tea **+** an orange slice **=** a strong but slightly sweet alternative to coffee with sugar

HEALTH BONUS: Black tea may help ward off Parkinson's disease, according to a study in the *American Journal of Epidemiology*. Eat the orange for a kick of vitamin C.

Green tea **+** a mint sprig **=** a heady brew

HEALTH BONUS: Japanese researchers found that green tea may protect your gums. Mint may improve alertness, according to a separate study.

Oolong tea **+** a sliced apricot **+** a sliced peach **+** additional fresh fruit **=** sangria iced tea

HEALTH BONUS: Oolong tea contains fat-blocking antioxidants, say Japanese researchers, and the fresh fruit will provide fiber, vitamins, and lots of flavor.

Iced coffee

Research shows that coffee can help you fight off Alzheimer's disease, colon cancer, depression, and type 2 diabetes. Avoid the calorie-clogged options at the chain coffee vendors (hint: if your order reads like Willy Wonka's grocery list, it's probably fattening), and go with straight unsweetened coffee, iced, with milk.

Flavored water

If you hate the taste of water, spruce it up. Keep a big pitcher in the fridge stuffed with ice and your own added ingredients to boost both the flavors and the visual appeal. That way, you'll always have an ice-cold, refreshing, beautiful beverage awaiting you every time you open the fridge. Going back to the artificial, metallic taste of the soda can would be a shame.

TRY

Ice water **+** a sliced lemon **+** a sliced lime **=** hint-of-citrus water

Ice water **+** a sliced orange **+** a sliced kiwifruit **+** the seeds from one pomegranate **=** tropics-tinged water

Ice water **+** slightly smashed blueberries **+** slightly smashed raspberries **+** slightly smashed blackberries **=** berry, berry good water

Ice water **+** a mango in chunks **+** three or four mint sprigs **=** mango-mint water

Other options at the grocery store:

Poland Spring Sparkling Water with Lemon Essence
Kick your soda cravings with this carbonated bottle that contains a hint of flavoring but no sugar. In fact, any seltzer at the store will do; just make sure it has no natural or artificial sweeteners, and you're safe.

R.W. Knudsen Sparkling Essence Lemon
Nothing in here but fizz, water, and lemon extract.

Hint Hibiscus Vanilla Essence Water
Hint's whole line of no-calorie, no-sugar flavored waters don't overpower—hence the name. Their peppermint and pear versions are good as well.

Izze Esque Sparkling Black Raspberry
If you can't shake your soda jones, at least pick a brand that doesn't use artificial ingredients. Izze's Esque line has half the calories of its other lines and still tastes great.

Skinny Swaps!

Swap good foods for bad, and you can lose weight the same way you gained it: Gradually. Consider these quick additions and substitutions to your menu.

DRINK EIGHT 8-OUNCE GLASSES OF ICE WATER

a day to burn nearly 500 extra calories a week. It takes about 3,500 calories to build a pound of fat—the amount that drinking this much ice water will save you in 7 weeks. Bottoms up! Good start!

SKIP THE SOFT DRINKS

High fructose corn syrup—the stuff that makes soda sweet—is more likely to be stored as fat than burned for energy, and it doesn't trigger the release of leptin, the hormone that stifles a raging appetite.

EAT WHOLE-GRAIN CEREALS

Australian researchers found that a daily bowl of refined cereal (i.e. with added sugars and refined grains) can raise your levels of insulin (a risk factor for diabetes) and C-reactive protein (a marker for inflammation) and lower your good cholesterol. A better choice: Post Shredded Wheat.

EAT THIS SWEET

Sweet potatoes have more fiber, and fewer carbs, than white potatoes, and they may help you look younger, longer. European researchers have found that the rich orange pigment builds up in your skin and prevents UV rays from making you look old before your time.

INCLUDE PROTEIN IN EVERY MEAL AND SNACK

Your gut has to work overtime to process it, so it takes twice as many calories to digest as other foods. Double bonus: It's the building block of muscle, so it'll help you beat the natural muscle-wasting effect of aging, as well.

REPLACE FRUIT JUICES WITH WHOLE FRUITS

If you eat the whole fruit, you eat more fiber and fewer calories than if you drink fruit juices— even those with lots of pulp.

EAT A HANDFUL OF DRY-ROASTED, UNSALTED NUTS EVERY DAY

It can lower your heart-disease risk by a third, chop your Alzheimer's risk by two-thirds, help reduce your blood pressure (and stroke risk) in stressful situations, and help you slim down.

EAT MORE BERRIES

Cranberries, blueberries, strawberries, and raspberries are all packed with antioxidants, which offer protection from stroke, keep you mentally sharp as you age, and help ward off cancer. Buy 'em by the bagful in the frozen-foods department and add them to yogurt, smoothies, and fruit salads, and to your ice cream bowl to take up space.

DOUSE YOUR SALAD WITH OIL AND VINEGAR

Unheated olive oil reduces cancer risk, and vinegar slows the absorption of carbs into your bloodstream—if you eat it early in the meal.

DOLE OUT DINNER, THEN STOW THE LEFTOVERS

If you leave serving platters on the table, you'll consume more calories than if you put them out of sight, back in the kitchen or fridge.

The Lean Belly Prescription Kitchen Makeover

Your supermarket carries 46,000 products, and not one of them can make it home without you. So be sure you bring home only the best foods. This swap 'n' shop guide will help you do it right.

STOCK YOUR KITCHEN, CHANGE YOUR LIFE

GIVE YOUR FRIDGE, FREEZER, AND PANTRY COMPLETE MAKEOVERS TO EAT HEALTHIER, COOK BETTER, AND START LIVING THE SKINNY LIFESTYLE YOU WANT TODAY.

Making healthy decisions has never been harder. Half the ingredients on food labels sound like your high-school chemistry homework. So-called healthy foods hide their secrets in tiny print on the backs of the packages. Refined foods strip essential vitamins and minerals from perfectly good whole foods, only to replace them with extra sodium, sugar, and calories. I hear your hardship, and I'm here to help.

Follow this better-foods buyer's guide to rid your kitchen of stuff that's been clogging your fridge, pantry, and arteries for years. Make the changes a few at a time, and you'll start eating better, losing weight, and living a healthier life.

Refrigerator Swaps
THE DOOR

Egg whites ➡ eggs

TRY Eggland's Best Grade AA Eggs, Extra Large

Per egg: 70 calories, 6 grams (g) protein, 4 g fat

Whole eggs are a great source of protein, and they contain more essential vitamins and minerals per calorie than virtually any other food. Plus, they are one of the best sources of choline, a substance that your body requires to break down fat for energy. Eggland's version has similar amounts of calories, fat, and protein as other brands, but with three times as many heart-healthy omega-3 fatty acids.

Margarine ➡ butter

TRY Keller's Whipped Butter, Salted

Per tablespoon (Tbsp): 70 calories, 7 g fat

Research shows that the fat in a pat of butter helps you better absorb vitamins A, D, E, and K. This brand cuts calories without sacrificing flavor.

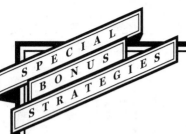
Regular ketchup ➡ organic ketchup

TRY Heinz Organic

Per Tbsp: 20 calories, 5 g carbs

Organic ketchups may have double the amount of prostate cancer-fighting lycopene that regular ketchups do. Plus, I think some brands' organic options—like Heinz's—taste better than the originals.

Regular mayo ➡ reduced-fat mayo

TRY Kraft with Olive Oil Reduced Fat

Per Tbsp: 45 calories, 2 g carbs, 4 g fat

Fat is not an enemy, but its calories add up quickly in mayonnaise. This mayo from Kraft has about half the calories of traditional versions, plus heart-healthy olive oil.

Dijon mustard ➡ regular mustard

TRY Annie's Naturals Organic Honey Mustard

Per teaspoon (tsp): 10 calories, 2 g carbs

Mustards tend to have few calories in the first place, but Dijon tends to have more sodium.

Regular beer ➡ light beer

TRY Coors Light

Per 12 ounces (oz): 104 calories, 5 g carbs

Standard brews can be heavy—some varieties have more than 200 calories per bottle. But by simply switching to the light version, you can often cut the calories by one-third.

THE DELI DRAWER

Bologna ➡ turkey

TRY Applegate Farms Organic Roasted Turkey Breast

Per 2 oz: 50 calories, 10 g protein, 1 g carbs

One slice of turkey has 6 grams of belly-filling protein—that's about double the amount in bologna. What's more, turkey contains only 22 calories per slice, compared to bologna's 57 calories. That's no baloney!

Salami ➡ ham

TRY Hormel Black Forest Ham

Per 2 oz: 60 calories, 9 g protein, 1 g carbs, 2 g fat

Salami packs 2½ times more calories than ham, almost 50 percent more sodium, and four times more fat.

American ➡ mozzarella

TRY Kraft Natural 2% Milk Mozzarella

Per oz: 70 calories, 8 g protein, 1 g carbs, 4 g fat

Reduced-fat mozzarella contains more protein than American, meaning your stomach will be satiated for much longer—one of the keys to losing weight.

Provolone ➡ Swiss

TRY Sargento Deli Style Sliced Reduced Fat Swiss

Per slice: 60 calories, 7 g protein, 1 g carbs, 4 g fat

One slice of provolone usually contains the same number of calories as a slice of Swiss, but it's not worth the extra 180 milligrams of sodium. Plus, Swiss contains an extra gram of protein compared with provolone.

Regular hot dogs ➡ smarter hot dogs

TRY **Applegate Farms Organic Uncured Beef Hot Dogs**
Per frank: 70 calories, 6 g protein, 4.5 g fat

Your typical hot dogs contain about 150 calories each. Applegate Farms' version cuts that number in half. Apply mustard and onions liberally.

THE SHELVES

Whole or fat-free milk ➡ 2% milk

TRY **Organic Valley Reduced Fat 2%**
Per cup: 130 calories, 8 g protein, 13 g carbs, 5 g fat

A little fat in your milk may help you absorb vitamins. The switch from whole moo juice to 2%, however, will save you 20 calories per cup.

Regular vegetable juice ➡ low-sodium vegetable juice

TRY **V8 Low Sodium**
Per 8 oz: 50 calories, 10 g carbs

Vegetable juice is a great idea if you struggle to meet the USDA's daily produce recommendation. The low-sodium V8 version has about one-fourth the sodium of the original vegetable juice, and it tastes better.

Orange soda ➡ orange juice

TRY **Tropicana Pure Premium Calcium + Vitamin D**
Per 8 oz: 110 calories, 26 g carbs

Think of it as a lesson in making calories count: Orange juice contains as many calories as a can of soda, but it also packs in essential vitamins and minerals. Even better, dilute your juices with one-half water to add more hydration and fewer calories.

Fat-free cottage cheese ➡ cottage cheese with some fat

TRY **Friendship 4% California Style**
Per ½ cup: 120 calories, 15 g protein, 3 g carbs, 5 g fat

Fat-free cottage cheeses contain close to 8 grams of carbs, but regular varieties tend to have less. So if you're eating it as a stand-alone snack, don't fear the extra grams of fat, which will help stabilize blood sugar. Friendship's cottage cheese has half the carbs of the competition's and a few extra grams of protein.

Fruity yogurt ➡ plain Greek yogurt

TRY **Stonyfield Farm Oikos Organic Plain Greek Yogurt**
Per 5.3-oz container: 80 calories, 15 g protein

Fruit varieties have more added sugars than plain yogurt does. I've seen some that contain as much as 36 grams! Greek yogurt brands like Oikos contain less sugar and more protein. If you miss the sweetness, stir in some fresh berries to replace that syrupy goop.

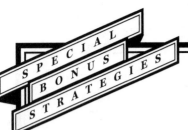
Sweet tea ➤ high-antioxidant tea

TRY **Honest Tea Organic Honey Green Tea**

Per 8 fluid (fl) oz: 35 calories

It's time to junk the sugar water. Green tea is known to pack a high nutritional punch, but in general, you want to look for a type with high levels of catechins—powerful antioxidants that could prevent disease. Honest Tea's offering has more catechins than its competitors'.

Soda ➤ sparkling water

TRY **Poland Spring Sparkling Water with Lemon Essence**

Per 8 fl oz: 0 calories

Sparkling water has all the bubbles of soda, without a single calorie. Flavored varieties are slightly sweetened. Make this change today and start shedding pounds.

THE CRISPER

There's really no such thing as unhealthy produce, so here are a few items to add to your refrigerator. Comparing what we actually eat to what Dietary Guidelines for Americans recommends, we consume less than half of the fruit we should and only 60 percent of the vegetables. Expand your tastes to include these, and improve your diet.

Vegetables

Beets
Although I personally don't like the taste of beets (so you won't find them in my crisper) this root vegetable is one of the best sources of folate and betaine—two nutrients that can decrease your risk of heart disease.

Lentils
These legumes have 16 grams of belly-filling fiber in every cup. What's more, compared to the same amount of cooked spinach, cooked lentils contain 27 percent more folate, which keeps your cells healthy.

Celery
Eating just four celery sticks a day can reduce blood pressure—sometimes by about 6 points on the systolic reading and 3 points on the diastolic.

Fruits

Blueberries
These berries, especially the wild ones, have more disease-fighting antioxidants than most other fruits.

Figs
This fruit is packed with potassium, manganese, and antioxidants, which makes it a potent immunity booster. The fiber from figs may also help lower insulin and blood sugar levels, reducing the risk of diabetes. Note that we aren't talking fig cookies here!

Grapes
Red grapes contain a potent antioxidant called resveratrol, which is believed to help fight cancer and heart disease—and even aging.

Freezer Swaps

We all have days when we just want to grab something from the freezer to mindlessly make for dinner. When this happens, you can avoid belly builders by strategically stocking your freezer.

Regular bean burritos ➽ chicken and bean burritos

TRY **Evol Burritos Cilantro Lime Chicken burrito**

Per burrito: 320 calories, 16 g protein, 49 g carbs (4 g fiber), 7 g fat

Chicken adds protein. Cilantro and lime add flavor—something you've probably never tasted with your usual bean burrito. Top with chopped tomatoes and shredded lettuce for an instant lunch or dinner.

Breaded frozen fish ➽ grilled frozen fish fillets

TRY **Gorton's Grilled Fillets, All Natural Lemon Butter**

Per fillet: 100 calories, 17 g protein, 1 g carbs, 3 g fat

Many times, "crispy" and "crunchy" are code words for "extra calories." The grilled version contains many fewer calories, with a hefty portion of protein.

Breaded chicken meals ➽ saucy chicken meals

TRY **Kashi Red Curry Chicken**

Per serving: 300 calories, 18 g protein, 40 g carbs (5 g fiber), 9 g fat

The extra calories that come in the breading aren't worth it—especially when you can replace empty calories with full-flavor ones. The double bonus here: The combo of kale, bok choy, and sweet potatoes adds a nice payload of fiber, as well.

Refined-grain pasta meals ➽ whole-grain pasta meals

TRY **Kashi Pesto Pasta Primavera frozen entrée**

Per meal: 290 calories, 11 g protein, 37 g carbs (7 g fiber), 11 g fat

All of your pastas, like your breads, should be whole grain. The extra fiber in whole grains helps you eat less at each meal. This Kashi entrée will fill you up, but won't overload you with calories.

Bagels and cream cheese ➽ Canadian bacon and egg sandwich

TRY **Jimmy Dean D-Lights Canadian Bacon Honey Wheat Muffin**

Per sandwich: 230 calories, 15 g protein, 30 g carbs (2 g fiber), 4.5 g fat

The protein in the sandwich will keep you fuller than the carbs in the bagel, making this a better option for breakfast to prevent gut grumbling until lunch.

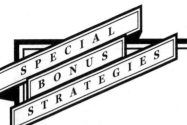

Regular french fries ➼ trans fat-free french fries

TRY Cascadian Farm Crinkle Cut French Fries

Per 18 pieces: 110 calories, 2 g protein, 17 g carbs (2 g fiber), 4 g fat

French fries have a bad rep—for a good reason. Some fries contain trans fats, a cheap, artery-clogging version of its heart-healthy mono- and polyunsaturated cousins. This brand is one of the few national brands that leaves out trans fats.

Regular ice cream ➼ low–fat ice cream

TRY Breyers All Natural Smooth and Dreamy Creamy Vanilla

Per ½ cup: 110 calories, 3 g protein, 16 g carbs, 3.5 g fat

Cut out sweets completely and you'll drive yourself diet-delirious. It's fine to treat yourself every now and then. This brand provides incredible taste, without a crushing number of calories.

Ice cream bars and sandwiches ➼ frozen fruit bars

TRY Edy's Fruit Bars

Per bar: 60 calories, 13 g carbs

Fruit bars normally contain fewer calories and less sugar than ice cream bars. The best brands, like Edy's, contain real fruit.

Regular pizzas ➼ thin-crust pizzas

TRY Palermo's Primo Thin Ultra-Thin Crust Pizza Special Edition Pepperoni frozen pizza

Per ⅓ pizza: 380 calories, 18 g protein, 24 g carbs, 23 g fat

Thin crusts slash calories and carbs, not flavor. As a rule, thin-crust varieties are healthier than deep-dish pizzas.

Regular waffles ➼ multi-grain waffles

TRY Van's 8 Whole Grains

Per 2 waffles: 180 calories, 3 g protein, 31 g carbs (6 g fiber), 7 g fat

This brand contains the valuable vitamins, minerals, and fiber that are stripped from refined grains. Sweetened with a touch of honey, they taste great, too.

Pantry Swaps

Kids' cereals ➤ whole-grain cereals

TRY **Kashi Whole Wheat Biscuits, Cinnamon Harvest**

Per 1.9 oz (28 biscuits): 180 calories, 6 g protein, 43 g carbs (5 g fiber), 1 g fat

Some cereals contain as much sugar as a scoop of ice cream. This brand still tastes sweet, but doesn't clobber you with simple sugars.

White bread ➤ whole-wheat bread

TRY **Arnold Grains and More Bread, Ancient Grains**

Per slice: 110 calories, 5 g protein, 21 g carbs (3 g fiber), 1.5 g fat

Make switching to whole-wheat bread one of the primary goals of your new diet. Whole grains provide vital fiber, vitamins, and minerals that refined grains don't. If you're worried about taste, Arnold Grains and More products taste amazing.

White flour ➤ whole-wheat flour

TRY **King Arthur White Whole Wheat**

Per ¼ cup: 100 calories, 4 g protein, 18 g carbs (3 g fiber), 0.5 g fat

You might as well bake with the stuff, too. Whole-wheat flour contains fiber and vitamin E—an antioxidant that reduces the risk of heart disease.

White rice ➤ brown rice

TRY **Uncle Ben's Ready Rice, Whole Grain Brown**

Per cup: 240 calories, 5 g protein, 39 g carbs (2 g fiber), 3 g fat

One ingredient: 100 percent whole-grain rice (plus a little healthy canola or sunflower oil for cooking). Uncle Ben's Ready Rice is ready to eat in 90 seconds.

Instant oatmeal ➤ steel-cut oatmeal

TRY **Arrowhead Mills Organic Steel Cut Oats Hot Cereal**

Per ¼ cup: 160 calories, 6 g protein, 27 g carbs (8 g fiber), 3 g fat

Steel cut oats contain more belly-filling soluble fiber—sometimes more than twice the amount, as is the case with Arrowhead's oats—than instant rolled oats.

Bagels ➤ English muffins

TRY **Rudi's Organic Bakery Whole Grain Wheat English Muffins**

Per muffin: 120 calories, 5 g protein, 23 g carbs (3 g fiber), 1 g fat

Think of English muffins as a thinner version of bagels—you'll shrink calories and carbs.

White pasta to ➤ whole-wheat pasta

TRY **Bionaturae Organic Whole Wheat Spaghetti**

Per 2 oz: 180 calories, 7 g protein, 35 g carbs (6 g fiber), 1.5 g fat

Are you sick of me with the whole grains yet? Don't worry, this pasta's so good, you barely need sauce.

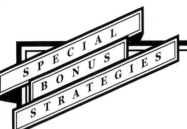

Vegetable oil ➤ canola oil

Vegetable oil is fine, but it's loaded with a lot of omega-6s and fewer omega-3s. Canola oil, on the other hand, has a near-perfect balance of the two fatty acids, which may help lower your risk of a variety of cardio-vascular ailments.

Peanut butter with trans fats ➤ trans fat–free peanut butter

TRY **Peanut Butter & Co. Crunch Time**
Per 2 Tbsp: 180 calories, 7 g protein, 8 g carbs (2 g fiber), 15 g fat

Look on the label of your PB: If it contains partially hydrogenated oil, change brands. Trans fats play with your cholesterol levels for the worse. Go with this pick, or narrow down your options by looking at the ingre-dient list—it only takes one to make peanut butter: peanuts.

Milk chocolate ➤ dark chocolate

TRY **Dagoba Beaucoup Berries Bar**
Per bar: 250 calories, 5 g protein, 27 g carbs (7 g fiber), 19 g fat

Pick chocolate with at least 65 percent cacao—the higher the per-centage, the higher the number of disease-fighting antioxidants. That being said, it should taste good, too, like this bar does.

High-sugar snack bars ➤ low-sugar bars

TRY **Lärabar Cashew Cookie**
Per bar: 230 calories, 6 g protein, 23 g carbs (4 g fiber), 13 g fat

The lower the sugar and the fewer ingredients on the label, the better. You want a quick pick-me-up, not a glorified candy bar. This brand has two ingredients: cashews and dates.

Potato chips ➤ low-calorie popcorn

TRY **Wise Choices Premium Pop-corn, Reduced Fat White Cheddar**
Per 3 cups: 140 calories, 3 g protein, 18 g carbs (3 g fiber), 6 g fat

Popcorn can be a surprisingly healthy snack—if it's the right kind. That's because it can leave you feeling full, without overloading you with calories. And don't forget to look for the trans fat–free kind.

Instant soup ➤ real soup

TRY **Lucini Italia Rustic Italian Minestrone Soup**
Per cup: 160 calories, 5 g protein, 22 g carbs (4 g fiber), 7 g fat

Forget ramen. Fill up on soups that contain doses of protein and fiber. This brand is filled with chunks of hearty vegetables—that don't require boiling water to reconstitute.

ARRANGE YOUR FRIDGE

You can change your diet by rearranging your refrigerator, as well. How you position your groceries shapes the way you eat and will help you reshape your belly.

Shelve strategically

Fill your eye-level shelf (or top shelf) with fruits, vegetables, and other nutritious snacks. You're 2.7 times more likely to eat healthy food if it's in your line of sight, a Cornell University study says. "That's also why manufacturers pay a premium to have their products at eye level in stores," says Kit Yarrow, Ph.D., a professor of psychology and marketing at Golden Gate University in San Francisco.

Pack smart

A variety of small containers with leftovers tempt you to eat more than you plan to, says Brian Wansink, Ph.D., author of *Mindless Eating: Why We Eat More Than We Think*. Instead, combine leftover entrées and sides so each container has one meal's worth.

Hide the junk

All stocked up on snacks? Now, place the healthy stuff front and center, and stash small guilty pleasures out of sight. In a 2009 Danish study, one in four participants who chose a healthy snack over an unhealthy one later reached for the junk anyway.

Shop more, buy less

Instead of hoarding supplies for the month, hit the supermarket more often and buy for only this week's meals. An overload of choices at home may deplete your willpower, a 2008 *Journal of Consumer Psychology* study found. "People tend to reduce consumption when resources are scarce," Yarrow says. Trick yourself into thinking it's a lean time and you'll become leaner.

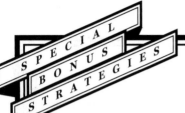
STEP THREE

BOOST FLAVOR, BLAST FAT

THESE INSTANT FLAVOR UPGRADES CAN
TRANSFORM YOUR MEALS AND SHRINK YOUR BELLY

Check out the nutritional information at most restaurant chains and you'll quickly learn their secret ingredients: calorie-clogged sauces and heavy doses of sodium. Don't follow suit. You can enhance the taste of home-cooked meals with these 10 quick and healthy flavor boosters.

Citrus

If you've ever squeezed a lemon wedge over fresh fish, you already know the power citrus holds. The acid in a lemon can brighten seafood, but it can also cut the heft of foods with natural fat. Try a squeeze of lime over your next round of steak tacos and note the difference. A few drops of a citrus fruit like a lemon, lime, or orange also tastes great squeezed into an ice-cold glass of water, spritzed across a fresh salad, or sprayed atop steamed vegetables as a no-calorie butter replacement.

Balsamic vinegar

This Italian staple has an acidity similar to that of citrus, but a flavor that's deeper and more complex. It's great for mixing with extra-virgin olive oil, fresh chopped herbs, mustard, salt, and pepper for an instant vinaigrette. Or, drip a few drops—balsamic vinegar is potent—over a grilled steak, sautéed greens, or, if you're feeling adventurous, a bowl of fresh berries. Trust me, you won't go back to chocolate syrup.

Herbs

Nothing compares to the aromatic flavors of freshly picked parsley, cilantro, basil, chives, thyme, sage, oregano, and rosemary. Add chopped herbs to eggs, pasta, soups, stews, or almost anything as a garnish. Your food will pop with color and disease-fighting antioxidants, too.

Marinades

These flavor baths amp up the taste of meats, poultry, seafood, and vegetables. Skip the boring stuff in the bottle and make your own instead. It's easy. The best marinades consist of three parts: acids (citrus, wine, plain yogurt), flavor builders (olive oil, mustard, honey), and accents (fresh herbs, spices, brown sugar). Mix and match these three components to suit your taste and soak your protein for a minimum of 30 minutes before grilling, or overnight for best results.

Salsa

It's not just for chips. Salsa makes the perfect vegetable-packed topping for foods fresh off the grill, especially fish and chicken. It also works well folded into an omelet for a south-of-the-border start to your day. Or, sauté some salsa with a can of black beans for a simple side dish.

Caramelized onions

They're sweet, savory, and delicious. Caramelized onions act as the perfect stand-in for higher-calorie mayo or dressing on burgers. To taste their full

power, try them atop a grilled steak or inside an omelet.
TO MAKE THEM: Heat 1 tablespoon of butter in a large saucepan over medium-low heat. Add four sliced red onions and a few pinches of salt, and cook until the onions have gone from translucent to a light caramel color, about 20 to 30 minutes. Then, add 2 tablespoons of balsamic vinegar and a few pinches of ground black pepper. Cook for 3 to 5 more minutes. It'll make a big batch, so keep the leftovers in the refrigerator. They'll keep for 10 days.

Wine

You love to drink it. You'll love to cook with it, too. Substitute white wine for water when steaming seafood for an instant flavor upgrade. Or add some red wine to a slow-cooked braise to intensify the deep, rich flavors of red meat. Whether cooking or sipping, price doesn't matter. The best rule is to cook with what you drink. If you like $8 chardonnay, cook with it. Then pour it at the table, and you'll have

created a quick harmony for the palate.

Olive oil

The hype is true. Olive oil is loaded with polyphenols—antioxidants that may help fight cancer, osteoporosis, and brain deterioration. Plus, olive oil is packed with heart-healthy monounsaturated fats. Choose extra-virgin olive oil, which has the highest polyphenol concentration. Pricey olive oil should be saved for dressing salads and vegetables. Regular or light olive oil is best for cooking.

Pepper and kosher salt

You can add as much pepper as you want, but be careful with salt. We get way too much sodium in our diets already (one reason a third of us have high blood pressure). To avoid a sodium overload, ditch the shaker. Pinch kosher salt straight from a dish. The coarse grains and the touch of your fingers give you maximum control. Add a pinch and taste, so you don't overdo it.

CHAPTER 5

Perfect Lean Belly Foods

Fuel your weight loss with tasty and healthy breakfasts, lunches, dinners, and snacks!

~~~~~~~~~~~~~~~~~~~~~~~~~~~~~~~~~~~~

O ne night recently, I took a break from working on this book to gas up the car for an upcoming trip. So as I drove to my local station, my thoughts were on fuel—the kind that propels you through life, and the kind you need on the interstate highway system.

I filled the tank, and then walked into the convenience store to pick up a few things—some milk, a packet of nuts for a snack, and other approved foods from my own personal PICK 3 TO LEAN shopping list. And that's when I saw a guy who I sincerely hope will read this book, some day.

Using my professional eye, I estimated his weight to be around 300 pounds. When I see a big guy, I see somebody who, all too soon, I'll probably meet in the E.R. I watched as he grabbed two extra-large Red Bulls, a liter of Mountain Dew, and a dozen doughnuts for good measure. He completed his purchases in front of the hot dog roller griller—hey, they looked enticing to me, too—walking away with a neat little box of them, at only 99¢ each.

All I could think was, "Good luck with all that, buddy. I'll be seein' ya (in the E.R.)."

I felt sad that night as I walked the aisles, looking at all the convenient, lousy food that people have come to view as "standard." What they don't see—what the guy in the store didn't understand, clearly—was that "standard" outcomes come from eating "standard" food. For two-thirds of us, that means being overweight or obese.

And that "standard" also leads inevitably to this part of my workday: "Dr. Travis," the nurse will tell me, "the patient in room 5 is an obese diabetic with kidney failure, and we think he's having a heart attack."

I'll grab the chart, look at the guy's medical problems, and think: "This was probably caused by an addiction to processed, carbonated crapola." The kind stocked on most of the shelves of this convenience store, in fact.

It doesn't have to be that way.

CHAPTER
5

LAWS OF
LEANNESS

You can enjoy your life more and weigh less—at the same time.

Whole foods fill you up without filling you out.

PRESCRIPTION MEALS FOR A MONTH

In the pages that follow, I'm giving you a week-by-week food plan that you'll enjoy and that will get you started on the road to a leaner life. I'm rewarding your willingness to experiment with change by suggesting awesome foods your tongue and belly will thank you for. After 4 weeks, many of these life-changers will become habits that help you lose fat as effortlessly as you gained it.

I'm providing you with 4 weeks' worth of meal plans for dinner Sunday through Thursday and lunches for the following days. (Take a look at dinner and lunch recipes together; sometimes you'll need to reserve some dinner leftovers, or else you'll be going without lunch the day after!) Fridays and Saturdays, you're more likely to be eating out or with friends, but you should apply the same principles: Eat whole foods, go for flavor over calorie count, and watch your portions. You should make it safely to Sunday, when the good home-cooked dinners begin again in week 2.

What many of us see as "standard" food is very unhealthy.	Big flavor means you won't miss big calories.	Cooking it yourself can save you time, money, and unnecessary pounds.	Food is the fuel that determines how well your engine runs.

Shop Once, Eat for a Week

Transforming your life means transforming your grocery list, too. That's why I'm supplying shopping lists (and recipes) to get you started. It's the beginning of an exciting time for you: identifying new foods and flavors you love, while breaking old habits that only got you into trouble. But that's my favorite way to solve a problem: Eat your way out of it. Enjoy!

Here is a balance of protein-packed meats, poultry, and seafood; fresh produce; dairy products; and a few versatile extras to feed yourself well, week after week.

THE PANTRY LIST

Before your first trip to the supermarket, check to see that you have these crucial flavor building blocks on your kitchen shelves. Restock every couple of months and you'll always have them on hand to construct meals around the clock.

For the REFRIGERATOR

- Cheese, Parmesan
- Eggs
- Mayonnaise, reduced-fat
- Mustard
- Pesto, basil, 1 jar (8 ounces)
- Pesto, sun-dried-tomato, 1 jar (8 ounces)
- Salsa
- Tomato paste, in a tube
- Worcestershire sauce

For the CABINET

- Basil, dried
- Blackening spice
- Chili powder
- Cinnamon, ground
- Cooking spray
- Cumin, ground
- Garlic, 4 bulbs
- Honey
- Hot-pepper sauce
- Molasses, mild
- Oil, canola
- Oil, olive, extra-virgin
- Onions, red, 2
- Onions, yellow, 2 pounds
- Peanut butter
- Peanuts, unsalted dry-roasted
- Pepper, ground black
- Red-pepper flakes
- Rice, brown, instant, 1 pound
- Sage, dried
- Salt
- Soy sauce, low-sodium
- Thyme, dried
- Vinegar, balsamic

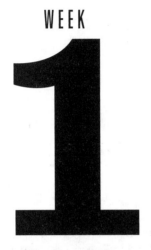
PRESCRIPTION GROCERY LIST

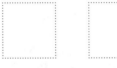

PRODUCE

- ☐ Asparagus, 1 bunch
- ☐ Avocado, 1
- ☐ Baby mixed greens, 4 ounces
- ☐ Bell peppers (1 red, 1 green, and 1 orange)
- ☐ Mushrooms, portobello, large caps, 2

PROTEIN

- ☐ Chicken, cooked rotisserie, 1 (about 3½ pounds)
- ☐ Pork, tenderloin, 1 herb-flavored or lemon-garlic marinated (about ¾ pound)
- ☐ Shrimp, frozen uncooked, medium, peeled, 1¼ pounds

DAIRY

- ☐ Cheese, mozzarella, shredded, 1 bag (8 ounces)

PACKAGED FOODS

- ☐ Beans, black, 1 can (12 ounces)
- ☐ Fettuccine, whole-wheat, 1 package (1 pound)
- ☐ Tortillas, whole-wheat (10" diameter), 1 package

✳ *All dinner recipes serve two. Lunches serve one. With a little experimentation, you should be able to adjust the portions for a family of three or four, or for when your friends note how lean and satisfied you are and beg for an invite.*

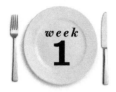

week
1

Chicken and Vegetables, Stat!

WHAT YOU'LL NEED

¾ bunch asparagus (about 8 spears), ends trimmed

2 portobello mushroom caps, sliced ¼" thick

1 onion, sliced ¼" thick

½ tablespoon + a drizzle extra-virgin olive oil

Salt

Ground black pepper

1 rotisserie chicken (about 3½ pounds)

1½ ounces (1½ cups) mixed greens

Balsamic vinegar

HOW TO MAKE IT

Preheat the oven to 400°F. In a baking dish, toss the asparagus, mushrooms, and onion with ½ tablespoon oil. Season to taste with salt and pepper.

Roast for 12 to 15 minutes, or until the vegetables are lightly browned.

Meanwhile, remove the skin from the chicken and discard. Use a fork to pull the meat from the bones. Reserve both breasts to serve with the roast vegetables. (It can be placed in the pan with the vegetables, if desired, to reheat during the last 4 minutes of roasting.) Place the remaining chicken on a cutting board and cut it into bite-size pieces—it should yield about 2 cups. Transfer the chopped chicken to an airtight container and refrigerate.

When the vegetables are cooked, reserve half of them. (After they cool, transfer to an airtight container and refrigerate.)

Serve the remaining vegetables with the reserved chicken breasts. Prepare a mixed-greens salad drizzled with oil and vinegar.

It's a (Chicken) Wrap!

HOW TO MAKE IT

Chop the peppers into ½" pieces. They should yield about 4 cups. Set ½ cup aside. Transfer 3½ cups to an airtight container and refrigerate.

In a small bowl, mix the mayonnaise, garlic, and vinegar. Brush the tortilla with the mixture. Sprinkle the cheese in a line down the middle, followed by the greens, chicken, and all the vegetables. To make a tight wrap, fold about ½" of the tortilla up first and then roll it from the side.

WHAT YOU'LL NEED

- 3 bell peppers (1 each of green, orange, and red)
- 1 tablespoon reduced-fat mayonnaise
- 1 clove garlic, minced
- 1 teaspoon balsamic vinegar
- 1 whole-wheat tortilla (10" diameter)
- 2 tablespoons shredded mozzarella cheese
- ½ ounce (about ½ cup) mixed greens
- ½ cup leftover chopped rotisserie chicken
- 1 cup leftover roasted vegetables

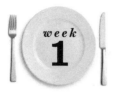

MONDAY'S DINNER

Nashville Shrimp Sizzle

WHAT YOU'LL NEED

¼ cup instant brown rice

1 avocado

½ can black beans, rinsed and drained, heated

½ tablespoon canola oil

1 onion, sliced

1 cup leftover chopped bell peppers

2 cloves garlic, minced

½ pound frozen uncooked, medium, peeled shrimp, thawed

½ teaspoon ground cumin

Red-pepper flakes or hot-pepper sauce

Salt

Ground black pepper

1 whole-wheat tortilla (10" diameter), warmed

HOW TO MAKE IT

Cook the rice according to the package directions.

Meanwhile, wash the avocado and with a small knife, cut it in half lengthwise, leaving the pit in one half. Tightly cover the half with the pit with plastic wrap. Refrigerate. Reserve the other half.

When the rice is cooked, add the beans. Heat the oil in a large skillet or wok over high heat. Add the onion, bell peppers, and garlic. Cook, tossing, for 5 to 7 minutes, or until the vegetables start to brown. Mix in the shrimp and cumin. Season to taste with red-pepper flakes or hot-pepper sauce, salt, and black pepper. Cook for 3 minutes, or until the shrimp are opaque.

Spoon half of the shrimp mixture on a plate with half of the rice and beans. Thinly slice the reserved avocado half. Add to the plate. Serve with the tortilla.

Reserve the remaining shrimp mixture with the rice and beans in a microwaveable bowl or plastic container for Tuesday's lunch.

NOTE: Makes 1 serving

Rice Bowl Rx

HOW TO MAKE IT

In a microwaveable bowl, warm the leftover Nashville Shrimp Sizzle in a microwave oven on high power for 1 minute, or until heated through. Top with the avocado and season to taste with salsa.

WHAT YOU'LL NEED

Leftover Shrimp Sizzle with rice and beans

Leftover ½ avocado, peeled, pitted, and thinly sliced

Salsa

Primetime Pasta

HOW TO MAKE IT

Cook the fettuccine according to package directions. Drain. Transfer half of the fettuccine to a storage container or resealable plastic bag. Drizzle lightly with oil. Toss to coat. Allow to cool and then refrigerate.

Return the remaining fettuccine to the cooking pot. Add the chicken, vegetables, and pesto. Toss to coat the fettuccine evenly. Season to taste with salt and pepper. Grate some Parmesan and sprinkle on top.

Prepare a mixed-greens salad drizzled with balsamic vinegar to taste.

NOTE: Makes 1 serving

WHAT YOU'LL NEED

6 ounces whole-wheat fettuccine

Extra-virgin olive oil

1 cup leftover chopped rotisserie chicken

1 cup leftover roasted vegetables

1½ tablespoons sun-dried-tomato pesto

Salt

Ground black pepper

Parmesan cheese

1½ ounces (1½ cups) mixed greens

Balsamic vinegar

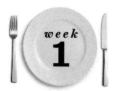

week
1

Q-Rating Quesadilla

WHAT YOU'LL NEED

- 1 whole-wheat tortilla (10" diameter)
- 1 tablespoon sun-dried-tomato pesto
- ½ cup (2 ounces) shredded mozzarella cheese
- ½ cup leftover chopped rotisserie chicken
- 1 cup leftover roasted vegetables

HOW TO MAKE IT

Place the tortilla on a microwaveable plate. Spread with the pesto. Top with the cheese, chicken, and vegetables. Heat in the microwave on high power for 1 minute, or until the cheese melts. Fold over and slice into quarters.

For a crispier result, cook the tortilla in a skillet over low heat.

As-Seen-on-TV Shrimp

HOW TO MAKE IT

Cook the rice according to the package directions.

Add the oil to a large skillet or wok and place over high heat. When the oil is smoking, add the bell peppers, asparagus, onion, and garlic. Stir-fry for 5 minutes, or until the vegetables are slightly browned. Stir in the shrimp and soy sauce. Cook, tossing, for an additional 3 minutes, or until the shrimp are opaque. Season to taste with hot-pepper sauce, salt, and black pepper. Transfer 1 cup of the mixture into an airtight storage container. Cool and then refrigerate.

Serve the remaining stir-fry over the rice.

WHAT YOU'LL NEED

½ cup instant brown rice

1 teaspoon canola oil

1 cup leftover chopped bell peppers

1 cup chopped asparagus

½ onion, chopped

2 cloves garlic, minced

¾ pound frozen uncooked, medium, peeled shrimp, thawed

1 tablespoon low-sodium soy sauce

Hot-pepper sauce

Salt

Ground black pepper

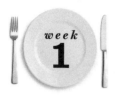

THURSDAY'S LUNCH

Broadcast Noodles #1: Thai Peanut

WHAT YOU'LL NEED

1 tablespoon peanut butter

½ tablespoon low-sodium soy sauce

1 tablespoon water

1 teaspoon balsamic vinegar

¼ teaspoon ground black pepper

1 cup leftover As-Seen-on-TV-Shrimp

3 ounces leftover cooked whole-wheat fettuccine

Hot-pepper sauce

1 tablespoon chopped unsalted dry-roasted peanuts

HOW TO MAKE IT

In a mixing bowl, whisk the peanut butter, soy sauce, water, vinegar, and black pepper until smooth. Add the stir-fry and pasta, tossing to mix thoroughly. Season to taste with hot-pepper sauce. Sprinkle on the peanuts. Eat cold or at room temperature.

Pork à la Stork

HOW TO MAKE IT

Preheat the oven to 450°F. In a baking dish, toss together the pork, onion, bell peppers, garlic, oil, and vinegar. Season to taste with black pepper. Bake for 20 to 25 minutes, or until a thermometer inserted in the center registers 155°F and the juices run clear. Let stand for 10 minutes before slicing.

Enjoy half the pork and vegetables tonight, and save the rest—storing both together in a sealed container— for lunch tomorrow. (If you want a bigger meal, re-heat the remaining whole-wheat fettuccine.)

WHAT YOU'LL NEED

1 herb-flavored or lemon-garlic mari-nated pork tender-loin, about ¾ pound

1 onion, quartered

1½ cups leftover chopped mixed bell peppers

2 cloves garlic, minced

1 tablespoon extra-virgin olive oil

1 tablespoon balsamic vinegar

Ground black pepper

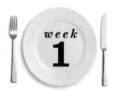

FRIDAY'S LUNCH

It's a (Pork) Wrap!

WHAT YOU'LL NEED

½ tablespoon sun-dried-tomato pesto

½ tablespoon reduced-fat mayonnaise

1 whole-wheat tortilla (10" diameter)

Leftover Pork à la Stork

2 tablespoons shredded mozzarella cheese

HOW TO MAKE IT

In a small bowl, combine the pesto and mayonnaise. Lay the tortilla on a plate. Spread on the pesto mixture. Thinly slice the pork. Layer the cheese, pork slices, peppers, and onions. Roll into a bundle.

WHAT ABOUT BREAKFAST?

I'm not going to make this too complicated, because who has much time first thing in the morning? Instead, let me give you some great quick-and-easy options, and you can choose among them. The key thing: Promise me you'll eat breakfast, or you'll spend the entire day filling that emptiness in your belly with foods you should be avoiding. Fill that void early, and for a long time, by eating protein, fiber, and fat within an hour of your wake-up time. To add a touch of sweetness, choose whole fruits or berries instead of fruit juice; you'll cut calories and add fiber. Suddenly, the wait for lunch got a lot shorter.

WAKE-UP WEIGHT-LOSS ALL-STARS

2 eggs, 2 strips of bacon, 1 slice of whole-wheat toast

Fruit smoothie (½ cup blueberries, ½ banana, 2 tablespoons peanut butter, 2 tablespoons whey powder, 1 cup milk, and 1 cup water, blended until smooth)

Whole-wheat English muffin, toasted, with almond butter, plus a piece of fruit

Any whole-grain cereal with more fiber than sugar (check the label; Kashi GoLean and Post Grape Nuts qualify), milk, and berries

Cooked steel cut oats, milk, raisins, slivered almonds, and cinnamon

Cooked quinoa, milk, a pat of butter, blueberries or raspberries, and toasted walnuts

A fried egg on a toasted English muffin, with a slice of Canadian bacon and a slice of Swiss cheese

Omelet (or scrambled eggs) with ham, onions, mushrooms, and spinach, with a slice of cantaloupe on the side

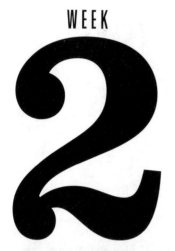

PRESCRIPTION GROCERY LIST

PRODUCE

- [ ] Arugula, 1 bag (6 ounces)
- [ ] Avocados, 2
- [ ] Broccoli rabe, 1 bunch
- [ ] Cabbage, red, 1 small head
- [ ] Celery, 1 bunch
- [ ] Cilantro, 1 bunch
- [ ] Lettuce, Boston, 1 head
- [ ] Limes, 4
- [ ] Mango, 1
- [ ] Pepper, green bell, 1
- [ ] Shallot, 1
- [ ] Thyme, 1 bunch
- [ ] Tomatoes, 2

PROTEIN

- [ ] Beef flank steak, 1½ pounds
- [ ] Chicken, thighs, bone-in, skinless, 4 (5 ounces each)
- [ ] Mahi mahi fillets, 2 (6 ounces each)
- [ ] Salmon fillets, preferably wild, 3 (4 ounces each)
- [ ] Turkey sausage links, lean Italian, 6 ounces

DAIRY

- [ ] Butter, salted, 1 stick (4 ounces)
- [ ] Yogurt, fat-free plain, 1 carton (6 ounces)

PACKAGED FOODS

- [ ] Bread rolls, whole-wheat, 2
- [ ] Chips, tortilla, 1 small bag
- [ ] Pasta, whole-wheat penne, 1 package (1 pound)
- [ ] Pita, whole-wheat, (6" diameter) 1 package
- [ ] Red wine, dry, half bottle (375 milliliters)
- [ ] Tomatoes, crushed, 1 can (15 ounces)

Stay-out-of-the-E.R. Salmon

HOW TO MAKE IT

Pour ½ cup of the wine into a saucepan. Recork the bottle and refrigerate.

Add the vinegar and shallot to the pan. Cook over medium-low heat for 10 minutes, or until the liquid is reduced by half. Remove from the heat to cool to room temperature. Add the butter, thyme, and a few pinches of pepper. Use a spatula to thoroughly mix the ingredients. Scoop the mixture onto a sheet of plastic wrap. Roll it up, twist the ends to form a log, and place in the freezer while you cook the fish. (You can prepare the wine butter in advance and refrigerate for up to 2 weeks.)

Coat a grill rack with cooking spray. Preheat the grill or grill pan.

Rub the salmon with oil. Season with salt and pepper. Lay the salmon, skin side down, on the grill or grill pan. Cook for 4 to 5 minutes, flip, and cook 2 to 3 minutes longer, or until the salmon is opaque.

Serve 2 of the fillets with a tablespoon of the red wine butter (reserve the remainder of each fillet in the refrigerator for another meal) on top. The heat of the fish fillet will melt it. Allow the remaining fillet to cool. Place in a small resealable plastic bag and refrigerate.

To make an easy side: Cut the tomato into six wedges. Divide between two salad plates and drizzle with oil. Season to taste with salt and pepper.

WHAT YOU'LL NEED

1 small bottle dry red wine (375 milliliters)

¼ cup balsamic vinegar

1 shallot, finely chopped

½ stick salted butter, at room temperature

1½ teaspoons fresh thyme leaves

Ground black pepper

3 salmon fillets (4 ounces each)

Extra-virgin olive oil

Salt

1 tomato

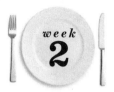

MONDAY'S LUNCH

Omega-3 Health-Wich

HOW TO MAKE IT

In a small bowl, combine 2 tablespoons reduced-fat mayonnaise, 2 teaspoons lime juice, ½ teaspoon minced garlic, and a sprinkling of chili powder. Stir to mix. Add a bit more lime juice to taste, if needed. Transfer half of the mayonnaise mixture to a small airtight container; refrigerate.

Spread the remaining mayonnaise mixture on a split whole-wheat roll. Top with last night's leftover grilled salmon, plus a leaf of Boston lettuce and a thick tomato slice.

Bachelor Balsamic Flank Steak

HOW TO MAKE IT

Jab the steak with a big fork in several places to create holes for the marinade to seep in. In a large resealable plastic bag, combine the vinegar, oil, pepper, and garlic. Set aside ¼ cup. Drop the steak into the bag. Seal the bag and massage to coat the steak. Put the bag in the refrigerator for at least an hour, or overnight.

Coat a grill rack or grill pan with cooking spray. Preheat to medium. Remove the steak from the marinade and grill, basting occasionally with the reserved marinade, for about 6 minutes per side or until a thermometer inserted in sideways in the center registers 145°F for medium-rare. Let stand for 10 minutes before slicing.

Slice the meat diagonally across the grain in thin slices. Transfer ½ cup of the meat to a resealable plastic bag; refrigerate. If you loved the wine butter from Sunday's dinner, serve some of it with the steak.

WHAT YOU'LL NEED

1 beef flank steak, about 1 ½ pounds

⅔ cup balsamic vinegar

¼ cup extra-virgin olive oil

1 tablespoon ground black pepper

3 cloves garlic, minced

week
2

Doctor's Orders Steak Salad

WHAT YOU'LL NEED

2 tablespoons extra-virgin olive oil

1 tablespoon balsamic vinegar

½ cup leftover sliced Balsamic Flank Steak

½ green bell pepper, finely chopped

2 ribs celery, finely chopped

¼ onion, finely chopped

4 cups arugula

HOW TO MAKE IT

In a mixing bowl, whisk the oil and vinegar. Add the steak, pepper, celery, and onion. Toss. Scatter the arugula on a plate. Spoon the salad over the arugula.

Travis's Teriyaki Chicken

HOW TO MAKE IT

Coat a grill rack or broiler pan with cooking spray. Preheat the grill or broiler to high.

In a medium bowl, combine the soy sauce, honey, and tomato paste. Stir to mix. Add the chicken and turn to coat all surfaces. Place the chicken on the grill or in the broiler pan under the broiler. Grill for about 4 minutes or broil for about 10 minutes, until well browned on the bottom. Flip and grill for about 2 minutes or broil for about 4 minutes until a thermometer inserted in the thickest portion registers 170°F and the juices run clear. Set aside 1 thigh for tomorrow's lunch. Serve with ½ cup instant brown rice, cooked according to package instructions.

WHAT YOU'LL NEED

2 tablespoons low-sodium soy sauce

1½ tablespoons honey

1 tablespoon tomato paste

4 bone-in, skinless chicken thighs (about 5 ounces each)

Waist-Not, Want-Not Chicken Pita

HOW TO MAKE IT

Remove the bone from the leftover chicken thigh. Tear the chicken into strips. Cut a pita in half and open to form a pocket. Stuff with a leaf of Boston lettuce, a few tomato slices, and drizzle with the leftover chili-lime mayo, and add the chicken. Eat with a few celery sticks.

NOTE: Store the remaining pitas in the freezer.

week
2

Fish Tacos Fresh from the Doc

WHAT YOU'LL NEED

1 mango, peeled, pitted, and cubed

1 avocado, peeled, pitted, and cubed

½ red onion, finely chopped

1 handful fresh cilantro, chopped

Juice of 1 lime + 2 wedges

Salt

Ground black pepper

2 mahi mahi fillets (6 ounces each)

Canola oil

½ tablespoon blackening spice

2 whole-wheat tortillas (10" diameter)

1 cup thinly sliced red cabbage

HOW TO MAKE IT

Coat a grill rack with cooking spray. Preheat the grill to medium-high.

Meanwhile, make the mango salsa. In a bowl, combine the mango, avocado, onion, cilantro, and lime juice. Season to taste with salt and pepper. Set aside.

Lightly drizzle the fish with oil and rub on the blackening spice. Place the fish on the grill and cook for 4 minutes, or until browned on the bottom. Carefully flip the fish with a spatula and cook for another 4 minutes, or until the fish is opaque in the center. Remove. Before turning off the grill, warm the tortillas directly on the surface for 1 to 2 minutes.

Reserve half of a fillet. Divide the remaining fish evenly between the warm tortillas. Add the cabbage and a large spoonful of salsa on top of each. Fold the tortillas in half, and serve each with a wedge of lime.

Refrigerate the remaining salsa in an airtight container. Refrigerate the half of fillet in a resealable plastic bag.

It's a (Fish) Wrap!

In a bowl, combine the yogurt, lime juice, and pepper. Fill each lettuce leaf with half of the avocado. Top each with several chunks of mahi mahi. Drizzle each with half the yogurt sauce and sprinkle on the cabbage. Fold each leaf into a wrap, along with a few cucumber slices. Accompany with tortilla chips and the leftover salsa.

1 carton (6 ounces) fat-free plain yogurt

Juice of 2 limes

Ground black pepper

2 large leaves Boston lettuce

½ avocado, peeled, pitted, and chopped

Leftover grilled mahi mahi, cut into chunks

¼ cup thinly sliced red cabbage

Tortilla chips

Leftover mango-avocado salsa

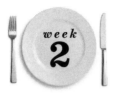

week
2

Broadcast Noodles #2:
Broccoli Rabe and Sausage

WHAT YOU'LL NEED

6 ounces lean Italian turkey sausage links (about 3 links)

1 tablespoon extra-virgin olive oil

¼ cup + 1 quart water

1 clove garlic, minced

1 can (15 ounces) crushed tomatoes

¼ teaspoon salt

8 ounces whole-wheat penne pasta

3 cups broccoli rabe, coarsely chopped

½ avocado, peeled and chopped

Boston lettuce, chopped

HOW TO MAKE IT

In a deep skillet, combine the sausage, oil, and ¼ cup water. Cover and cook over medium-high heat until the mixture simmers. Reduce the heat if needed and cook until the water evaporates.

Uncover the pan and continue cooking the sausage, turning as needed, for about 5 minutes, or until well browned. Remove the sausage. Cool 1 link and refrigerate in a resealable plastic bag for tomorrow's lunch. Cut the remaining sausage into ½"-thick slices.

Return the sausage to the pan with the garlic and broccoli rabe. Cook over medium-high heat for 1 to 2 minutes, or until the garlic is golden. Stir in the tomatoes. Cover partially and simmer over medium-low heat for 10 minutes until the flavors blend and the broccoli rabe is tender. Reserve ⅓ cup of the sauce, cooling it and then refrigerating it in an airtight container.

Bring a pot of salted water to a boil. Stir in the penne and cook according to packaging instructions. Drain, then combine with the sausage and broccoli rabe.

On the side, serve a simple salad of avocado and Boston lettuce.

Sausage: The Sequel

HOW TO MAKE IT

Heat the oil in a small skillet over medium-high heat. Add the pepper and onion. Cook, stirring occasionally, for 5 minutes or until golden. Stir in the leftover sausage and leftover tomato sauce. Simmer for 1 to 2 minutes to warm.

Split a toasted whole-wheat roll. Fill with the sausage mixture.

WHAT YOU'LL NEED

2 teaspoons extra-virgin olive oil

½ green bell pepper, thinly sliced

¼ onion, thinly sliced

Leftover turkey sausage link

Leftover tomato sauce

1 whole-wheat roll

Eat the Rainbow

The next time you visit the grocery store try to buy at least one piece of produce from every color of the rainbow. The Centers for Disease Control and Prevention confirms that it's a great way to take in a range of nutrients.

RED

Many red foods contain anthocyanins and lycopene, which may fight cancer. Others have potassium to control blood pressure and vitamin A to keep your eyes healthy.

Tomatoes

PEAK: June to September
PICK: Go for heavy ones with rich color and no wrinkles, cracks, bruises, or soft spots. They should have some give under light pressure from your fingertips.
STORE: Never in a fridge; cold destroys flavor and texture. Keep them out of direct sunlight for up to a week.
PAYOFF: Lycopene, to help you dodge heart disease, cancer, and macular degeneration

Strawberries

PEAK: April to September
PICK: Seek out unblemished berries with a bright-red color extending to the stem and a strong fruity smell. They should be neither hard nor mushy.
STORE: Place unwashed berries in a single layer on a paper towel in a covered container.
PAYOFF: The most vitamin C of all commonly eaten berries

Watermelon

PEAK: June to August
PICK: Pick it up; you want a dense melon free of cuts and sunken areas. The rind should be dull, with a creamy yellow underside. A slap should produce a hollow thump.
STORE: Keep whole in the fridge for up to a week to prevent the flesh from drying out and turning fibrous.
PAYOFF: Citrulline, an amino acid that can help improve blood flow

ORANGE

These are carotenoid-rich foods that are good sources of immunity-boosting vitamin A and vitamin C, which promote oral and overall health.

Peaches

PEAK: May to October
PICK: Good peaches have a fruity aroma and a yellow or warm cream background color, without green shoulders. They're ready when they yield to gentle pressure on the seams. And take a big whiff—the fragrance is one of the delights of fresh peaches!
STORE: Leave unripe ones out at room temperature. Ripe ones go in the fridge, but eat within 2 to 3 days.
PAYOFF: Vitamin C, beta-carotene, fiber, potassium

Papayas

PEAK: June to September
PICK: Look for papayas that are starting to turn yellow and yield a bit when lightly squeezed.
STORE: Once ripe, eat immediately or refrigerate for up to 3 days. Green

papayas should be ripened at room temperature in a dark setting until yellow blotches appear.
PAYOFF: Lots of fiber and vitamins A, C, E, and K

Produce of this color often contains vitamin C, which helps heal wounds and clears out disease-causing free radicals.

Pineapple

PEAK: March to July
PICK: Look for vibrant green leaves, a bit of softness to the fruit, and a sweet fragrance at the stem end. Avoid spongy fruit.
STORE: If it's unripe, keep it at room temp until it softens and gives off a pineapple aroma. Refrigerate for up to 5 days.
PAYOFF: Niacin for skin and gastrointestinal health, and manganese for bones

Bell peppers

PEAK: Year-round
PICK: These should have lots of heft for their size and sport brightly colored, wrinkle-free exteriors. The stems should be a lively green.
STORE: Refrigerate in the crisper for up to 2 weeks.
PAYOFF: All bell peppers are loaded with antioxidants, especially vitamin C. Yellow peppers lead the pack.

GREEN

These are good sources of magnesium, which helps to protect your bones. Some greens are rich in vitamin K, needed for proper blood clotting.

Broccoli

PEAK: October to April
PICK: Find rigid stems with tight floret clusters that are deep green or tinged with purple. Pass on any with yellowing heads—they'll be more bitter.
STORE: Refrigerate in a plastic bag for up to 1 week.
PAYOFF: Cancer-fighting sulforaphane

Asparagus

PEAK: February to June
PICK: Buy vibrant green spears with tight, purple-tinged buds. Thin spears are sweet and tender.
STORE: Trim off the woody ends. Stand the spears in a bit of water in a lidless tall container; cover the tops with a plastic bag. Cook within a few days.
PAYOFF: Folate, which may protect the heart and promote weight loss.

Kiwifruit

PEAK: Year-round
PICK: A ripe kiwi will slightly yield to the touch. Avoid mushy or wrinkled ones with an "off" smell.

STORE: Leave at room temperature to ripen. To quicken the process, place them in a paper bag with an apple or a ripe banana. Once ripe, refrigerate in a plastic bag for up to a week.
PAYOFF: 65 percent more vitamin C than in a small orange

BLUE & PURPLE

Produce of these colors usually house the anthocyanins that protect cells from oxidative damage.

Eggplant

PEAK: August to September
PICK: It should feel heavy and have tight, shiny skin. When pressed, you want springy, not spongy.
STORE: Keep in a cool location (not the fridge) for up to 3 days.
PAYOFF: Chlorogenic acid, which grabs free radicals

Blueberries

PEAK: May to October
PICK: You want plump, uniform berries with taut skin and a dull white coating.
STORE: Transfer them unwashed to an airtight container and refrigerate for 5 to 7 days.
PAYOFF: More disease-fighting antioxidants than most common fruits

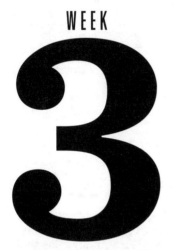

WEEK 3

PRESCRIPTION GROCERY LIST

PRODUCE

- [ ] Arugula, 1 bag (6 ounces)
- [ ] Basil, 1 bunch
- [ ] Lemon, 1
- [ ] Lettuce, romaine, 1 head
- [ ] Scallions, 1 bunch
- [ ] Tomatoes, 2

PROTEIN

- [ ] Beef sirloin or top round steak, ¾" thick, ½ pound
- [ ] Chicken breast halves, boneless, skinless, 3
- [ ] Pork tenderloin, 1 pound
- [ ] Shrimp, frozen uncooked, medium, peeled, ½ pound

DAIRY

- [ ] Cheese, blue, crumbled, 1 small container
- [ ] Cheese, mozzarella, shredded, 1 bag (8 ounces)
- [ ] Yogurt, fat-free plain, 1 carton (6 ounces)

PACKAGED FOODS

- [ ] Bread, sourdough, 1 small loaf
- [ ] Fettuccine pasta, whole-wheat, 1 package (1 pound)
- [ ] Whole-wheat flatbread, soft (7" diameter), 1 package
- [ ] Roasted red peppers, small jar
- [ ] Vegetables, frozen stir-fry mix, 2 bags (14 ounces)

Chat Show Chicken

HOW TO MAKE IT

Pierce each chicken breast in several places with a fork.

In a large resealable plastic bag, combine the oil, Worcestershire sauce, vinegar, garlic, honey, and basil. Add the chicken. Seal the bag and massage gently to coat the chicken. Marinate in the refrigerator for at least 30 minutes.

Coat a grill rack or grill pan with cooking spray. Preheat the grill to medium high heat.

Remove the chicken from the marinade. Grill the chicken for 10 minutes on each side, or until a thermometer inserted in the thickest portion registers 160°F and the juices run clear. Set aside 1 chicken breast. Cool and then refrigerate in a clean resealable plastic bag.

Serve with a salad of arugula and roasted red peppers drizzled with olive oil and balsamic vinegar.

WHAT YOU'LL NEED

3 boneless, skinless chicken breast halves

2 tablespoons extra-virgin olive oil + extra for drizzling

2 tablespoons Worcestershire sauce

2 tablespoons balsamic vinegar + extra for drizzling

3 cloves garlic, minced

1 tablespoon honey

2 teaspoons dried basil

2 ounces (2 cups) arugula

2 roasted red peppers, chopped

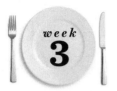

Prescription Panini

HOW TO MAKE IT

In a blender or food processor fitted with a metal blade, puree ¼ cup roasted red peppers with a little oil, vinegar, and salt. Smear the mixture on 2 slices toasted sourdough bread. Cut ½ leftover grilled chicken breast into thin diagonal slices. Lay on the bread. Top with some blue cheese crumbles and chopped arugula. Drizzle with balsamic vinegar.

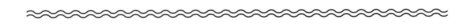

Paunch-Free Pizza

WHAT YOU'LL NEED

- 3 soft whole-wheat flatbreads (7" diameter)

- 2 tablespoons basil pesto

- 1 tomato, thinly sliced

- 1 small handful fresh basil leaves

- ¼ cup shredded mozzarella cheese

HOW TO MAKE IT

Preheat the oven to 425°F. Set the bread on a small baking sheet. Spread the pesto on the bread, dividing it evenly between the two. Add a layer of tomato and a layer of basil on each. Sprinkle half of the cheese over each. Bake for 7 minutes, or until the cheese is golden and melted. Set aside 1 pizza. Cool and wrap in aluminum foil. Refrigerate.

Cold-Case Pizza

Cut the remaining leftover ½ grilled chicken breast into thin diagonal slices. Fan out over the leftover pizza, and top with a few arugula leaves.

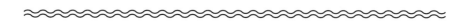

Broadcast Noodles #3: Grilled Shrimp

In a large resealable plastic bag, combine the shrimp, lemon juice, and garlic. Seal and massage gently to coat the shrimp. Refrigerate for 15 minutes, turning occasionally.

Coat a grill rack or grill pan with cooking spray. Preheat the grill or grill pan to medium high heat.

Drain the marinade into a 10" skillet. Set aside the shrimp. Over medium heat, bring the marinade to a boil. Add the peppers and scallions. Cook, stirring occasionally, for 2 to 3 minutes or until all the liquid has evaporated. Remove from the heat. Add the pesto, yogurt, and lemon peel.

Cook the pasta according to package directions. Drain and add to the skillet.

Grill the shrimp for 2 minutes on each side, or until opaque. Set aside about one-quarter of the shrimp, allowing it to cool. Then transfer it to a resealable plastic bag and refrigerate. Add the remaining shrimp to the skillet. Toss to mix the ingredients. Serve with lemon wedges.

- 1 pound frozen uncooked medium shrimp, peeled and thawed
- 2 tablespoons lemon juice
- 6 cloves garlic, minced
- ⅓ cup roasted red peppers
- ¼ cup chopped scallions
- ¼ cup basil pesto
- ¼ cup fat-free plain yogurt
- 1 teaspoon grated lemon peel
- ½ pound whole-wheat fettuccine

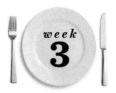

WEDNESDAY'S LUNCH

It's an (Asian Shrimp) Wrap !

HOW TO MAKE IT

In a small bowl, combine 1 tablespoon peanut butter with a splash of low-sodium soy sauce and 1 teaspoon honey. Stir until smooth. On a piece of soft flatbread, spread the peanut butter and layer some chopped scallions and a leaf of romaine. Add the leftover grilled shrimp. Roll it up.

WEDNESDAY'S DINNER

Stork Pork 'n Herbs

WHAT YOU'LL NEED

- ¾ pound pork tenderloin
- 2 teaspoons extra-virgin olive oil
- ½ teaspoon crumbled dried sage
- ½ teaspoon dried thyme
- 1 small clove garlic, minced
- ¼ teaspoon salt
- ¼ teaspoon ground black pepper

HOW TO MAKE IT

Preheat the oven to 375°F. Cover a shallow baking dish with aluminum foil and place the pork on it. Drizzle the oil over the pork. Sprinkle on the sage, thyme, garlic, salt, and pepper. Rub to coat the pork evenly with the seasonings.

Roast for 30 to 35 minutes, or until an instant-read thermometer inserted in the center registers 155°F and the juices run clear. Let stand for 10 minutes before cutting into thin slices.

Pack about one-fourth of the pork into a small resealable plastic bag. Refrigerate.

Stork Porkwich

HOW TO MAKE IT

Spread 2 slices sourdough bread with a thick slather of pesto and a few fresh basil leaves. Top with the leftover pork. Add a shower of mozzarella cheese and close the sandwich. Microwave until warm.

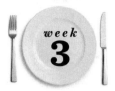

THURSDAY'S DINNER

Belly-Off Asian Beef

WHAT YOU'LL NEED

- ½ cup instant brown rice
- 1 beef sirloin or top round steak, about ½ pound, thinly sliced
- 2 tablespoons low-sodium soy sauce
- 2 teaspoons canola oil
- 1 bag (14 ounces) frozen stir-fry vegetables, thawed
- 2 cloves garlic, minced
- ½ cup diagonally sliced scallions
- ¼ cup coarsely chopped unsalted dry-roasted peanuts

HOW TO MAKE IT

Cook the rice according to the package directions.

In a bowl, toss the meat with 1 tablespoon soy sauce. Set a wok or large skillet over high heat for 1 minute. Add the oil. Swirl to coat the pan. Place the meat in a single layer in the pan. Cook, without stirring, for about 1 minute, or until browned on the bottom. Stir. Cook 1 minute, stirring once or twice, until no pink remains. With a slotted spoon or tongs, transfer the meat to a dish and set it aside. Pack about one-eighth of the meat into a small resealable plastic bag. Allow to cool and then refrigerate.

Add the vegetables to the pan. Stir-fry over medium heat for about 5 minutes, or until the vegetables are heated. Add the garlic. Stir-fry for 30 seconds. Add the reserved meat, rice, scallions, peanuts, and the remaining 1 tablespoon soy sauce. Toss for about 1 minute until heated.

Green Room Salad

In a large bowl, combine the lettuce, beef, tomato, scallions, and garlic. Drizzle lightly with oil. Toss well to coat. Top with the cheese.

2 ounces (2 cups) chopped romaine lettuce

Leftover Asian Beef

1 tomato, chopped

2 tablespoons scallions, chopped

1 small clove garlic, minced

Extra-virgin olive oil

3 tablespoons blue cheese crumbles

HIGH ENERGY WITHOUT HIGH CARBS

SKIP THE ENERGY SHOTS AND POWER BARS—
USE REAL FOODS TO FUEL YOUR BRAIN AND BODY

Yes, technically all foods containing calories give you energy, even a chocolate doughnut. But if you want lasting energy—energy that chocolate doughnut can't provide—you'll need to stick to real foods. Here are six to start you off and power you through.

Peanut butter

Beyond PB's ability to help your heart, prevent Alzheimer's, and deliver antioxidants, it's also an excellent source of protein. Remember we are talking pure peanut butter here, not the kind with added sugar. One tablespoon carries 4 grams of protein for only about 90 calories, most from healthy monounsaturated fats. Go ahead, spoon it out of the jar as a snack. Tell them Dr. Travis told you to do it.

Hard-boiled eggs

These awesome ovals are one of nature's perfect energy boosters. Eggs contain a bevy of important vitamins and minerals, and egg whites are one of the purest forms of protein available in whole foods—exactly what you'll need to feed your muscles after a workout.

Chocolate milk

You heard correctly. A glass of this delicious moo juice provides the carbohydrate-to-protein balance your muscles need to recover quickly from exercise and keep you energized throughout the rest of your day.

Raspberries

Bursting with antioxidants, fiber, manganese, and vitamin C, these little berries will keep your heart and brain in top shape. Try them blended into a smoothie, tossed with a fresh blue cheese and spinach salad, or straight out of the container as a snack.

Bananas

No wonder marathon runners love this fruit. Its potassium aids muscle movement, its fiber fills you up, and its good carbohydrates keep you energized. Not to mention that a banana is the perfect on-the-go snack—it's already in its package! In fact, I think I may just have one right now!

Oatmeal

Oats contain plenty of fiber and complex carbohydrates. Complex carbs fill you up by providing nice, even blood sugar levels instead of the spikes you'd feel from eating quick-digesting simple carbs. Whip up a batch in the morning, or heck, anytime, adding fresh fruit or a little cinnamon.

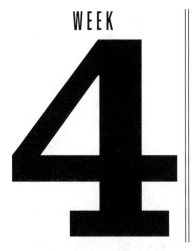

WEEK 4

PRESCRIPTION GROCERY LIST

PRODUCE

- Bok choy, baby, ¾ pound
- Mushrooms, brown, 12
- Spinach, baby, 3 bags (6 ounces each)
- Tomatoes, cherry, 1 carton
- Zucchini, 1

PROTEIN

- Bacon, 1 package (½ pound)
- Beef, ground, 93% lean, ½ pound
- Beef, London broil, about 1" thick, 1 pound
- Lamb, boneless, shoulder or leg, 12 ounces
- Scallops, sea, 8, ½ pound
- Tilapia fillets, ¾ pound

DAIRY

- Cheese, mozzarella, shredded, 1 bag (8 ounces)
- Cheese, ricotta, 1 container (15 ounces)
- Eggs, 1 carton (half dozen)

PACKAGED FOODS

- Bread roll, ciabatta, 1
- Chicken broth, 12 ounces
- Coffee, ground or instant
- Couscous, whole-wheat, 1 box (7 ounces)
- Pasta, whole-wheat penne, 1 package (16 ounces)
- Sesame seeds, small container
- Tomatoes, diced, 2 cans (15 ounces each)

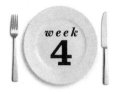

week
4

Star-Quality Scallops

WHAT YOU'LL NEED

8 sea scallops
(½ pound)

¼ teaspoon salt

1 egg, beaten

¼ cup sesame seeds

1 tablespoon canola
oil

¾ pound baby bok
choy, quartered
lengthwise

HOW TO MAKE IT

Set a steamer basket in a saucepan filled with about 2" water. Cover and set over medium heat.

Pat the scallops dry and season both sides with salt. Encrust each scallop on one side by dipping that side into the beaten egg and placing it on a plate spread with the sesame seeds.

Heat the oil in a 12" skillet over medium heat. Place the scallops, sesame-seed side down, in the skillet, leaving space between them. Cook for 3 to 4 minutes, until the seeds are golden. Flip each scallop carefully and cook for another 6 minutes, or until opaque. Cool 2 scallops and pack in an airtight container to refrigerate.

Meanwhile, when the water boils, put the bok choy in the steamer basket. Cover and steam for 6 minutes, or until just tender. Serve the remaining scallops nestled among the bok choy quarters.

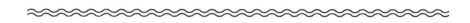

New Leaf Spinach Salad

HOW TO MAKE IT

In a small skillet, fry 2 slices bacon until crisp. Drain on paper towels. In a salad bowl, combine 2 big handfuls spinach. Crumble on the bacon and drizzle with a little canola oil. Toss and transfer to a plate. Top with the leftover scallops.

Broadcast Noodles #4: Spicy Beef

HOW TO MAKE IT

Preheat the oven to 350°F. Coat an 11" x 7" baking dish with cooking spray.

Cook the penne according to package directions but 3 minutes less than the indicated cooking time, or until slightly underdone. Drain and rinse under cold water. Transfer one-quarter of the pasta to a large resealable plastic bag. Cool and refrigerate.

Heat a large nonstick skillet over medium-high heat. Crumble the beef into the pan. Cook, stirring with a wooden spoon to break up any chunks, for 3 to 4 minutes, or until no pink remains. Remove one-third of the beef and transfer to an airtight container. Cool and refrigerate.

Add the onion, garlic, basil, and red-pepper flakes to the skillet. Cook for 3 to 4 minutes, or until the onion starts to soften. Add the tomatoes, tomato paste, and salt. Stir and reduce the heat to medium. Simmer for about 10 minutes, or until slightly thickened.

Meanwhile, in a bowl, combine the ricotta cheese, ½ cup of the mozzarella cheese, and the Parmesan cheese.

Pour half of the penne into the bottom of the prepared baking dish. Top with half of the sauce. Dollop on the ricotta mixture. Top with the remaining penne and the remaining sauce. Sprinkle the remaining ¼ cup mozzarella over the top.

Bake for 30 minutes, or until the sauce bubbles and the cheese melts. Let stand for 5 minutes before serving.

WHAT YOU'LL NEED

- ½ pound whole-wheat penne pasta
- ½ pound 93% lean ground beef
- ½ cup chopped onion
- 2 cloves garlic, minced
- ½ teaspoon dried basil
- ¼ teaspoon red-pepper flakes
- 1 can (15 ounces) diced tomatoes
- 1 teaspoon tomato paste
- ¼ teaspoon salt
- ½ container (15 ounces) ricotta cheese
- ¾ cup shredded mozzarella cheese
- 1½ tablespoons grated Parmesan cheese

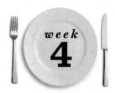

TUESDAY'S LUNCH

Skinny Steak Sandwich

HOW TO MAKE IT

Cut a thawed whole-wheat pita in half and open to form a pocket. Fill with ¼ cup shredded mozzarella cheese and leftover ground beef. Microwave on high power for 1 minute, or until warm. Season to taste with hot-pepper sauce, red-pepper flakes, or chopped scallions.

Fit Fillet, Mediterranean Style

HOW TO MAKE IT

Transfer one-third of the tomatoes and juice to a small bowl or jar. Cover tightly and refrigerate.

In a large skillet, heat the oil and garlic over medium heat for 2 minutes, or until fragrant. Add the broth, red-pepper flakes, salt, and remaining tomatoes with juice. Bring to a boil. Reduce the heat to a brisk simmer. Cook for 8 minutes, or until the mixture thickens.

Place the fish in the pan. Press lightly to submerge in the sauce. Cover and cook for 8 minutes, or until the fish flakes easily. Remove the fish to 2 pasta bowls. Add the spinach to the skillet. Increase the heat to high. Cook, stirring occasionally, for 2 minutes, or until the spinach is wilted. Spoon all but one-quarter of the spinach and tomato sauce over the fish. Pack the remaining sauce in an airtight container. Cool and refrigerate.

WHAT YOU'LL NEED

- 1 can (15 ounces) diced tomatoes
- 1 tablespoon extra-virgin olive oil
- 2 cloves garlic, minced
- ⅓ cup chicken broth
- ¼ teaspoon red-pepper flakes
- ¼ teaspoon salt
- 2 tilapia fillets
- 1 bag (6 ounces) baby spinach

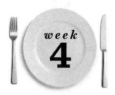

WEDNESDAY'S LUNCH

Broadcast Noodles #5:
Spinach and Tomato Sauce

HOW TO MAKE IT

In a microwaveable bowl, combine the leftover penne with the leftover spinach and tomato sauce. Stir. Cover and microwave on high power for 90 seconds, or until heated. Season with red-pepper flakes and a drizzle of olive oil.

Metabolic Beef Booster Shot

WHAT YOU'LL NEED

- 1 beef, London broil, 1" thick (about 1 pound)
- Coffee, ground or instant
- 1 tablespoon extra-virgin olive oil
- ½ onion, chopped
- 2 cloves garlic, minced
- ½ teaspoon red-pepper flakes
- ½ teaspoon ground cinnamon
- Leftover diced tomatoes
- ¼ cup Worcestershire sauce
- 1 tablespoon balsamic vinegar
- ¼ cup light molasses
- Salt
- Ground black pepper

HOW TO MAKE IT

Brew ¼ cup plain coffee or reconstitute instant coffee to make 1¼ cups. Cool.

In a large nonstick skillet, heat the oil over medium-high heat. Add the onion and garlic. Cook for about 2 minutes, or until softened. Add the red-pepper flakes and cinnamon. Cook for 1 minute longer. Pour the mixture into the bowl of a food processor fitted with a metal blade. Add the tomatoes, coffee, Worcestershire sauce, vinegar, and molasses. Process into a coarse puree. Return the mixture to the skillet. Season to taste with salt and black pepper. Bring to a simmer. Cook, stirring occasionally, for 15 to 20 minutes, or until thickened.

Meanwhile, preheat the broiler. Coat a broiler pan with cooking spray.

Place the beef on the pan. Brush one side with sauce and broil for 7 to 9 minutes, or until browned on top. Turn the meat over, brush with some more sauce, and cook for another 7 to 9 minutes for medium-rare (when a thermometer inserted in the center registers 145°F) or longer to desired doneness. Bring the remaining sauce in the skillet to a boil for 1 minute. Cut the meat into thin slices. Pack one-quarter of the meat into a resealable plastic bag. Cool and refrigerate. Serve the remaining meat with the extra sauce on the side.

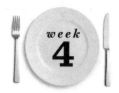

THURSDAY'S LUNCH

London Broil (On Hippocratic Loaf)

HOW TO MAKE IT

Split a ciabatta roll. Fill with leftover London Broil, a few spinach leaves, and a few shakes of hot-pepper sauce.

Lean-Belly Lamb Kebabs

WHAT YOU'LL NEED

3 tablespoons leftover dry red wine

3 teaspoons extra-virgin olive oil

4 cloves garlic, minced

12 ounces boneless lamb shoulder or leg, cut into cubes

1 zucchini, cut into cubes

12 brown mushrooms

1 onion, cut into 12 wedges

12 cherry tomatoes, halved

⅔ cup chicken broth or water

1 bag (6 ounces) spinach

HOW TO MAKE IT

In a large resealable plastic bag, combine the wine, 1 teaspoon of the oil, and half of the garlic. Add the lamb, zucchini, mushrooms, onion, and cherry tomatoes. Seal and massage gently to coat ingredients. Marinate for 20 minutes, or as long as 8 hours in the refrigerator.

Coat a grill rack with cooking spray. Preheat the grill.

Remove the lamb and vegetables from the marinade. Thread the lamb and vegetables, dividing evenly, onto 3 long skewers. Grill over medium heat, turning occasionally, for 10 minutes or until the meat is cooked to desired doneness.

Reserve 1 skewer and cool. Then remove the lamb and vegetables and pack into an airtight container. Refrigerate.

In a medium skillet, heat the remaining 2 teaspoons oil over medium heat. Add the remaining garlic. Cook for 1 minute, or until tender. Add the broth or water and the spinach. Cover and cook, stirring once, for 2 minutes, or until the spinach wilts. Sprinkle in the couscous. Stir. Cover the pan and turn off the heat. Allow to sit for 5 minutes or until the spinach wilts. Serve with the 2 kebabs.

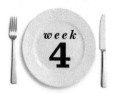

Doctor's (Lunch) Orders: Lamb Pita

HOW TO MAKE IT

Cut a thawed whole-wheat pita in half and open to form a pocket. Stuff with the leftover lamb and vegetables. Top with a mixture of equal parts reduced-fat mayonnaise and mustard. Eat with a handful of cherry tomatoes on the side.

What about Snacks?

One key to shrinking your belly is to fight off the food cravings that lead you to overeat. The best way to do that: Maintain consistent blood sugar levels with intelligent snacking between meals. Build your snacks using one protein + two other food groups, including a fruit or vegetable.

TRIM TRIOS THAT WORK

banana **+ almond butter** **+ milk**	**whole-grain crackers** **+ peanut butter** **+ celery sticks**	**whole-wheat tortilla** **+ turkey slices** **+ tomato**
dark chocolate **+ peanut butter** **+ apple**	**string cheese** **+ baby carrots** **+ hummus**	**black bean chips** **+ salsa** **+ Cheddar cheese**
strawberries **+ cottage cheese** **+ mixed nuts**	**orange** **+ Greek yogurt** **+ trail mix**	**mixed berries** **+ Greek yogurt** **+ walnuts**

Swap these choices around, and you have dozens of possibilities to tide you over from one meal to the next. When your belly grumbles, you can answer it.

Food Fixes!

What's the result of mindless eating? Endless weight gain. But if you give me 10 seconds, I'll give you ways to eat better and grow leaner at the same time.

CUT 3,500 CALORIES A WEEK, AND EAT BETTER

A study from the U.S. Department of Agriculture found that people eat an extra 500 calories a day when they hit the drive-through than when they prepare their own meals. The reason: Fast food tends to be high in calories, carbohydrates, sodium, and fat. Drive past the drive-thru, and you could easily avoid 3,500 calories a week—enough to lose a pound a week.

BUTTER, BETTER

It's a great source of conjugated linoleic acid, a potent fat fighter. Just don't go crazy; it has 102 calories per tablespoon.

NO-GO FISH?

A single ounce of walnuts has as many waist-trimming, brain-clearing, heart-helping omega-3 fatty acids as 4 ounces of salmon.

SCALE DOWN

Overweight people who weigh themselves at least once a week are six times more likely to lose weight.

SIX-MEAL SOLUTION

People who eat three meals and three snacks stoke their metabolism, making them half as likely to become overweight as people who eat three or fewer meals per day.

WHO CAN'T DO THAT?

Cut 96 calories from your daily diet and you could be 10 pounds lighter 1 year from today.

LOONEY-TOON NUTRITION

Almost 90% of the foods marketed to kids are lousy nutritionally. If the ad pitch comes from a cartoon character, be very, very suspicious.

SHOP ON WEDNESDAY

Only 11% of people do that, so the aisles will be clear and your choices will be better, especially in the the skinny sections of the supermarket: meat and fish departments, and produce.

IT'S PRONOUNCED KEEN-WA

The South American grain quinoa is classified as a carb, but it packs fiber, nutrients, and protein in abundance, as well. Cook it up with raisins, cinnamon, and (a little) maple syrup for breakfast.

WHY MR. PEANUT HAS A SKINNY WAIST

Swedish scientists had one group of people snack on 1,360 calories per week of candy, and another group snack on the same caloric payload of peanuts. After 2 weeks, the candy eaters gained weight and waist size. The peanut eaters just boosted their fat-burning metabolism.

HUNGER STOPPER

Eat extra protein for breakfast (eggs, bacon, Greek yogurt, milk, and cheese) and you'll stay extra full all day.

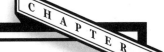
The 24-Hour Fat Burn

It's time to get reintroduced to the greatest fat-burning machine ever created: your body. Here's how to reprogram it to melt belly fat all day, every day!

~~~~~~

Y ou learn a lot about people when you work as an E.R. doctor. Emergencies can bring out the worst in them—and the best. Sometimes they're eager to fix the problem that landed them on the gurney, and sometimes they blame everybody but themselves for their presence there. The saddest cases: people who are so beaten down by their health woes that they can't muster much energy of any kind. They just accept the bad news, because recently, that's the only kind they hear.

Before I joined the faculty at Vanderbilt University Medical Center, I did a stint at a group of hospitals in central Colorado. There, I treated many patients who had been injured pursuing the sports they loved: skiing, mountain biking, hiking, rock climbing, running. These were active people, and they sometimes were beaten by a tough adversary: gravity. They'd fall, and they'd get scraped up, or they'd break a bone, and I'd help patch them back together.

You might be thinking, *Serves 'em right for doing all that dangerous stuff. Hope they learned a lesson.* But the number one question these active types would ask me was: "When can I get back on my bike/mountain/cliff face/skis/trails?" They could hardly imagine life without the activities that made their lives so enjoyable.

These people did suffer injuries, some of them serious. But because they were motivated to take care of themselves and were operating from a base of fitness and overall good health, they were usually able to bounce back, often stronger than they had been before their unfortunate run-ins with the ground.

Which brings me to my beloved Tennessee, which unfortunately has one of the highest rates of obesity in the country and where I've learned what the most dangerous activity of all is: none.

When I pull back the curtain in a hospital cubicle, I often find a patient who's at least 30 pounds overweight, dealing with a complication directly related to that excess weight.

And these self-inflicted injuries are usually more grievous than any that gravity can impose; when I patch up a fit, active person, he

---

CHAPTER
—— *6* ——

LAWS OF
LEANNESS

| The best exercise program in the world is the one you enjoy doing. | Find activities you love, and pursue them with people you love (or at least like pretty well). |

or she is often healed in a matter of days or weeks. When I patch up a person who's seriously overweight, he or she may never be fully healed. As I've said before, that's why I wrote *The Lean Belly Prescription*—because for every lean belly I can help shape, that's a life possibly saved or extended.

You've already learned some incredibly easy nutrition swaps, and gotten a bunch of great new foods and recipes to enjoy. But there's one more thing you need to do if you really want to turbocharge your weight loss.

You need to get active.

YOU CAN BURN CALORIES WITHOUT "WORKING OUT"

Too many Americans think exercise is for Michael Phelps and David Beckham, not for people like them. It's almost as if the running boom and the extreme-sports boom and the triathlon boom and the mountain-biking boom have convinced a lot of us that, if we're not willing to push it to an X Games level, we shouldn't bother exercising at all.

In fact, for the best workouts, you don't need much equipment at all—just your body and a willingness to put it in motion. And as you'll discover in this chapter, there are all sorts of ways to build more motion—and enjoyment, and companionship—into your life. And you don't have to lift a dumbbell or train for a 5-K to burn meaningful calories.

I know this is so, because I've seen convincing studies on non-exercise activity thermogenesis—a concept we'll explore in some detail.

You can burn more calories doing everyday activities than in workouts.	Schedule activity time every day.	To change your waist size, change speeds as you exercise.	Even 5 minutes is enough time to exercise. It all counts, it all adds up!

But I also know it from studying one particular lab rat: myself.

I learned the value of adding activity right after college, when I started my first career, as a financial analyst in Washington, D.C. I spent my days sitting at my desk crunching numbers, and found myself with nothing too exciting to do on the weekends other than watching some football on TV and drinking some beers with friends at night. Even in my early twenties, I was beginning to see changes in my body that I didn't like—long hours in a desk chair were not making me feel any younger! What I needed was to bring a little more balance to my life. So I went and bought myself a bicycle.

This won't be the last time you'll hear me talking about balance. It's the activity concept that works for all of us non-Armstrongs. Nobody's asking you to pedal to the top of the Alps in France. Instead, you simply need to balance your energy equation—good food in, good fun burning it off doing activities that you enjoy. Fat-burning shouldn't be a chore or an obligation, but a way of living your life to the fullest, of making time for the people and the activities that you love.

After I bought my bike, I started out riding on the weekends, and I found great routes through the surrounding area. I hadn't ridden a bike since elementary school, but in a few short months I became hooked. I lived for those bike rides and the change of scenery they gave me. Pretty soon I asked myself, *If I enjoy this so much on weekends, why not ride my bike to work?* So I became one of the few pedal-powered number crunchers in the Beltway area. Growing up in the Midwest, I had never even considered going to work in anything other than a car. But after I started commuting by bike, something funny happened. I started to look forward to getting up and going to work. I didn't love my job but I did love the commute.

My bike was carrying me toward new views and experiences, and I began to seek them out when I was out of the saddle, as well. That's how I started volunteering in a free clinic and an emergency room. I walked into the hospital thinking of myself as a "math guy," only to learn that my number skills were pretty pale stuff compared with the lifesaving talents of the people in surgical scrubs. They were quickly calling the shots and changing people's lives while they did it.

The more I watched the doctors fulfilling their life-altering mission, the more I thought that that's where I belonged in life, too. Eventually, I decided to quit my finance job and apply for medical school. My parents were pretty surprised. They'd thought they'd already settled me into the career that I'd pursue for a lifetime. Wasn't it risky to chuck all that and launch into a decade of medical training?

Yes, it was.

But the momentum I'd gained on my bicycle rides—improvising new routes and taking in amazing new perspectives—was now carrying me in whole new directions in my life. It was thrilling. And I can't help but think that the mental energy I'd added with my two-wheeled hobby was somehow spurring me onward toward new meaning in my life.

Could you use more of that spirit of discovery in your life? Then put more forward motion into it. There's a big world out there, and the most active people get to see more of it. That is one of the best lessons I've ever learned, and it didn't come from medical school.

A NEW WAY OF THINKING ABOUT EXERCISE

Here's a typical encounter with exercise, one that millions of Americans experience every year. See if it squares with what has happened to you. A woman proposes a new commitment to exercise to her husband, maybe as a joint New Year's resolution. He agrees, and they head off to Sears to drop $800 on a stairclimber or a tread-mill or an elliptical machine. They lug the thing into the basement—the dreariest place in the house, which is the only place they could agree to put a pretty ugly machine—and commit to a certain number of minutes a week on the thing. They start off strong, maybe even losing a few pounds. But they're not admitting the obvious thing to each other: It's boring to exercise by yourself in the basement, the view is lousy, and those 30 minutes are the longest of the day. Plus, it's lonely; instead of spending time with loved ones, they're off someplace else, alone. Pretty soon husband and wife hit busy times at work, or the kids land parts in the school play, and time is pinched. What is the first thing to go? The worst part of the day: exercising in the basement. Soon the stairclimber becomes a hanging rack for style mistakes bought on sale.

What went wrong? These well-meaning people fell victim to exercise hype, the idea that working out is a very complex process requiring expensive machines and commitments to fancy health clubs and hours and hours of sweating in front of wall-size mirrors. What kind of people want to live in their basements or look at themselves for hours in a gym? Not the kind I want to spend time with.

Who do I want to spend time with? My family and my friends, of course. You're probably the same way. If you can find active pursuits you enjoy and build your social and emotional lives around those activities, you'll lose weight while gaining more of what we all need in our lives: friendship and love.

So much of the research I've read about sticking with an exercise plan says that the most important factor in keeping fit is who you're exercising with, not what exercise you're doing. So you can see how the stairclimber in the basement falls short. Incorporating exercise into your social life often means setting weekly appointments for the walk or hike or bike ride. Or it can mean that you all commit to doing the charity walk and set a goal for yourselves to get ready for it.

The point of all of this: to find activities you love to do with people you love to be with. Then exercise becomes a reason for socializing, not a boring chore you'd do anything to avoid.

START BURNING FAT TODAY!

This starts what might technically be known as the "exercise" portion of the book, but I'd rather call it what it really is: the fun part of the book! Why? Because not everybody is cut out for what we usually think of as "exercise": hoisting barbells in the gym, or pounding out the miles on the road. And here's the shocker: You can burn far more calories just living your daily life than you ever could with scheduled gym sessions. In fact, the energy you burn in your everyday activities can boost your burn by as much as 2,000 calories each and every day! That's as true for people who avoid gyms as it is for 7-days-a-week exercisers.

Scientists call the regular-life calorie burn non-exercise activity thermogenesis (NEAT), but I prefer to think of it by a simpler name: having fun. I'll propose four ways to do that; pick one, and use it to add calorie-burning rocket fuel to the eating plan you designed for

Talk Yourself into Exercising

Turns out, some reasons are more persuasive than others, according to a study in the *Journal of Applied Biobehavioral Research*. The thoughts on the right are still great, but they might not propel you out the door!

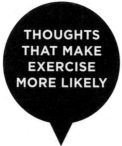

THOUGHTS THAT MAKE EXERCISE MORE LIKELY

I'll listen to music or a book, or watch TV, while working out

—

I'll exercise in a comfortable environment (like an air-conditioned, uncrowded gym)

—

I'll make a schedule

—

I'll make exercise interesting (like choosing a treadmill with a good view)

—

I'll set a goal

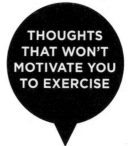

THOUGHTS THAT WON'T MOTIVATE YOU TO EXERCISE

I won't feel tense or like a failure

—

I'll have more energy

—

I won't be grumpy with other people

—

I'll set a good example for my kids or friends

—

I'll be in a better mood

yourself in Chapter 4 or the one I outlined in Chapter 5.

And if you've already started to eat healthier, you're going to find the suggestions in this chapter even easier to follow—and vice versa. Researchers at the University of Pittsburgh found that eating right encourages you to build more activity in your life, and more activity reminds you to eat better. When you do both of those things, you'll have written your own prescription weight-loss plan, based on foods you love and activities you already enjoy.

This won't be medicine you choke down; you can enjoy taking it. Feel free to increase the dosages whenever you want! The more Lean Living Turbochargers you choose, the more you lose!

"I love watching TV!"

I do too, and I'm glad you do, as well; my job as host of *The Doctors* depends on healthy people parking themselves in front of the tube, at least for part of the day! But I know that too much tube time can be a real drain on my system. According to a study done in Australia, overweight people spent 49 percent of their leisure time watching TV. Lean people spent only 28 percent of their leisure time in front of the TV. I've also seen an interesting study that showed that the negative effects of watching television for 1 hour can be counterbalanced by 30 minutes of exercise. And I live my life by that equation. That is, if I'm planning to spend 2 hours watching my alma mater (Duke) play another team from the ACC in basketball, I'll make sure I get in 1 hour of acivity that day. That's a lot, especially for new exercisers, and especially given how much TV the average American watches each day (about 5 hours' worth). So let me propose this: If you love watching TV, make a conscious decision to add activity to your day, to earn that sitting-downtime. Commit to 10 minutes of activity for every hour you watch. And it doesn't have to be all at once: A 20-minute walk at lunch, another after dinner, and 10 minutes of housecleaning or playing with the kids will do it. You'll have burned between 200 and 400 calories just by doing that (who needs a rowing machine?), and you can watch TV knowing that you've earned the right to heckle the contestants on *Dancing with the Stars!*

WHY YOU SHOULD DROP THE REMOTE

In a recent study, Australian scientists analyzed the leisure-time habits of more than 2,000 people. Their finding: The most sedentary Aussies were the most overweight, and they spent about 3 hours a day—almost 50 percent of their downtime—in front of a TV. (In the U.S., we average 5 hours!) The leanest, most active people watched the box for just 56 minutes.

PERCENTAGE OF LEISURE TIME SPENT BY:

Overweight sedentary people...		Lean active people...
49%	WATCHING TV	28%
8	USING THE COMPUTER	<1
1	PLAYING VIDEO GAMES	<1
12	READING	12
14	SITTING AND TALKING	12
15	DRIVING FOR LEISURE	12
1	BEING PHYSICALLY ACTIVE	35

"I love spending time with my family!"

Then by all means enlist them in the cause. In fact, their lives may depend on it. Researchers from the University of Alabama determined that a body mass index (BMI) of 25 to 35 can shorten a life by up to 3 years. So make weight loss a family affair. Sedentary men are 50 percent more likely to work out three times a week if they do it with their partners, according to a Duke University study. Of course, I define "work out" pretty broadly, to include scheduling a nightly walk after dinner, hikes or bike rides on the weekends, a couple of hours volunteering to clean up the yard around the church. I also define "family" loosely. For those social benefits of exercise, you can join a league or sign up for a team. A study in the *British Medical Journal* found that people who exercise in groups burn an average of 500 extra calories per week compared to those who exercise alone. Heck, even playing with the kids counts. According to a study published in the *Journal of Sports Medicine and Physical Fitness*, just 20 minutes of playing soccer or dodgeball raised adults' heartbeats to 88 percent of their maximum and burned 160 calories; half an hour burned 240 calories—about the same as a moderate bike ride. So if you love spending time with your family, exercising with them can build your relationships and shrink your belly at the same time. Just make sure the activity spikes happen on a regular schedule, and last long enough to fully engage you with the people in your life.

"I love a change of pace!"

Then have I got the "exercise" plan for you. It's called interval training, and you can apply its benefits to nearly any activity you enjoy. Simply change speeds or exertion levels, and you're a fat-burning inferno. Here's how it works. In an Australian study, people who cranked out 20 minutes of high-intensity interval training 3 days a week dropped 10 percent of their body fat, while those who exercised longer but at a lower intensity didn't lose any. If you've already invested in a gym or home exercise equipment, you can take advantage of the machines to beat boredom and ignite your weight loss by performing the study's exercise-bike routine: On a stationary bike, sprint for 8 seconds, then slow to an easy pace for 12 seconds. Repeat that back-and-forth for 5 minutes. Go for longer as the sessions become easier. But you don't have to do that. In fact, if you love a change of pace, you can apply the principle of interval training to nearly any activity. Go to page 146 for ideas. If you enjoy walking or biking, choose a hilly route, so that you'll have to work harder on the uphills, and you can catch a break on the downhills. If you live in a flat place, play the telephone-pole game: accelerate when you pass one, slow down when you pass the next. Or change pace with every mailbox, maple tree, or McMansion. This is the kind of cheating even a college professor can endorse: If you alternate between going hard and easing off, it all counts as "high-intensity training." Researchers in Virginia found that it significantly reduces total abdominal fat, abdominal subcutaneous fat, and abdominal visceral fat—disarming the murderer's row around your middle. If you want to change your waist size (for the smaller), change your exercise intensity as well.

"I love the idea of burning fat without any formal exercise plan!"

To know NEAT—non-exercise activity thermogenesis—is to love it. James Levine, M.D., at the Mayo Clinic, has studied this all-day energy burn, and he has determined that NEAT can account for as much as 50 percent of your metabolism—all through everyday movements.

He and his colleagues discovered this by wiring up people's underwear. That's right, they gave volunteers specially outfitted undies that could continuously monitor all kinds of movements they made during the day for 10 days. In the study, the leanest people burned 350 more calories per day than overweight people. Three hundred and fifty more calories a day, *without formally exercising*. Assuming you aren't David Copperfield, how do you pull off that magic trick?

You treat your whole life as your "workout," that's how. It doesn't need to be difficult, but you do need to seize opportunities to move your butt the way most of us—in this world of laborsaving devices— seize ways to remain on the couch. So if you love the idea of burning fat without any formal exercise plan, commit to the NEAT life. Stand up to take phone calls in your office. Walk down to your colleague's office rather than sending an e-mail. (Taking their own research to heart, Levine and his colleagues invented something they call the "walking meeting," where, instead of lounging around a conference room while they jaw, they stroll the halls of the Mayo Clinic instead.) Spend your lunch hour walking to buy a salad from a restaurant half a mile away, and eat it back at your desk.

If you're going to be watching the football game for 4 hours on Saturday afternoon, go out in the backyard and toss the ball around at halftime. And those chores you're avoiding? These four—ironing seven shirts, raking the leaves for 20 minutes, mopping the floors for 22 minutes, pulling weeds for 25 minutes—will burn 400 calories. (Giving your mate a 19-minute massage will burn a 100, so swap that in and maybe he/she will reciprocate!) You know your daily routine far better than I, but I'm certain there are lots of opportunities to add footsteps, add exertion, add purposeful movement, and see more of life at the same time. Here are some other simple ways to work NEAT into your life:

➜ Do you endlessly circle the parking lot outside the grocery store, looking for the closest parking space? Save time by choosing an empty space in the corner of the lot instead. And burn calories!

➜ When you step inside the mall, avoid the escalators, which are diabolical machines designed to build your love handles. Take the stairs instead, where the skinny people are elevating their fitness levels and themselves at the same time. And burn calories!

➜ Keep a Swiss ball in your family room, and spend 15 minutes out of each hour sitting on the thing, even if you're just watching the tube. You'll make subtle adjustments to maintain your balance, keep up with your favorite prime-time shows, and burn calories!

➜ Buy one of those electric toothbrushes with a built-in timer to make sure you brush for at least 2 minutes—it's the best thing for your oral health. But it's also incredibly boring. So while you brush, balance on one leg to engage the stabilizing muscles of your legs. Alternate legs when the toothbrush signals you to change regions of your mouth. You'll be more balanced, and burn calories!

➜ Hit the public walking trail. Scientists at the University of Utah observed that people who use public walking and cycling trails at least once a week are twice as likely to meet government exercise recommendations as those who don't. The researchers also found that lean people frequented the paths more often than heavyweights did. Seem like an obvious connection? It is. So do it. And burn calories!

➜ When you're staying at a hotel, by all means use the elevator when you check in with your luggage. Avoid it the rest of the time.

Weight Loss Made Simple

You know you should use the stairs, not the escalator. But while this advice may sound pat, heeding it can have a significant impact on your daily energy expenditure. Try the five simple strategies below and you will—almost effortlessly—stoke your metabolism and burn about 10 percent more calories a day.

	+ DO THIS	**–** NOT THIS	**=** EQUALS
1	Go for a brisk 20-minute walk	Sit for your entire lunch hour	**49 extra calories burned**
2	Stand during three 10-minute phone calls	Put your feet up on your desk	**33 extra calories burned**
3	Play vigorously with your kids or pets for 15 minutes	Watch TV before dinner	**82 extra calories burned**
4	Spend 15 minutes washing the dishes by hand	Head straight to the couch	**27 extra calories burned**
5	Take 10 minutes to straighten up one room	Go right to bed	**21 extra calories burned**

212 extra calories burned | All-day metabolism boost: 10 percent

Walking up the few flights might even save time over what you'd otherwise spend staring at the elevator door while you wait for it to come and then listening to elevator music. Burn calories instead!

→ Set an alarm on your computer to sound every 30 minutes. When you hear the tone, stand up and fetch a glass of ice water (drinking eight glasses of ice water will burn 64 calories a day), or simply stretch your arms over your head for 30 seconds. It breaks up motionless minutes and burns calories that would otherwise go to...waist.

→ Take your dog for a walk. Researchers at the University of Victoria in Canada found that people who own dogs walk almost twice as much as the dogless. It's because Fido's "parents" can't say no to the pooch, according to study author Ryan Rhodes, Ph.D. Pets are pushy. Doctors at Northwestern Memorial Hospital in Chicago discovered that when it comes to exercise, dogs are "consistent initiators." Dog owners exercise, on average, 132 minutes more each week than people who don't own dogs. Pick up the leash, and burn calories! No dog? What are you waiting for? Adopting a canine is like hiring a 24/7 trainer.

I can almost hear you thinking, *And you call this exercise, Dr. Travis?* Yes, I absolutely do, but I can see why you might not be convinced. We've all been conditioned to believe that "serious" exercise—and by that we mean counting the miles we've run or the iron we've pumped— is the only way to become fit. And I'm a big believer in traditional exercise—I've included a terrific workout plan in Chapter 7. But if you don't enjoy exercise, you don't need exercise. All you really need is *activity.*

THE SNEAKY WAYS
THAT FAT ATTACKS

Have you noticed that the more overweight our society gets, the more gyms open up? And the more gyms that open up, the fatter we all get? Why might that be?

Well, it doesn't mean that exercise makes us fat. But what it suggests is that the things we do when we're not exercising play a much bigger role in our weight than we might think. University of Minnesota scientists surveyed a group of people between 1980 and 2000, and the number who said they did some form of regular exercise stayed pretty consistent over those 2 decades. But the researchers were surprised to find that the same group spent about 8 percent more time sitting—at home, at work, in restaurants, in their cars.

Now we're getting to the bottom (and a big one it is) of the problem.

Compare that with how life was a couple hundred years ago, in our great-grandparents' day. Nobody had the luxury of sitting around because there was too much work to do. It turns out that some Dutch scientists have figured out exactly how much. They hired a group of actors to pretend to be Australian settlers for a week, doing all the activities that were necessary back then: foraging for food, chopping wood, scrubbing clothes. Then they compared the actors with a group of current-day office workers. Our 19th-century counterparts walked an average of 3 to 8 more miles *per day*—not to mention the calories they burned chopping and scrubbing.

I'm not suggesting that you sell your car and walk everywhere. But I am suggesting that the more activity you build into your day, the less you'll weigh, and the healthier and happier you'll be. According to one French study, the secret to losing your belly fat isn't how many calories you burn during formal exercise, but, rather, how much time you spend in motion. We're not talking about a world-record marathon pace here. Just simple movement, added wherever and whenever you can during the day. If you can add in 5 minutes here, 10 there, until you reach 4 more hours in motion per week, you'll join the population with the leanest midsections and probably book a beach vacation to show it off.

Think it's too late to start? I assure you, it isn't. A German study of 300 people determined that those who *started* getting more active in their forties were twice as likely to avoid heart disease compared with nonexercisers. That's nearly the same as the benefit enjoyed by people who have worked out for their entire lives.

So, if you're hankering to jump into a workout program, just turn the page. I've based *The Lean Belly Prescription* exercise regimen—I call it "The World's Easiest Exercise Plan"—on the latest weight-loss and fitness research. And it will turbocharge your weight loss like you won't believe. But if exercise just isn't your thing, don't worry: You don't need to go to the gym to start slimming down!

INTERVAL TRAINING FOR BEGINNERS

It sounds complicated and intimidating, right? But interval training has been shown to be the most efficient way to burn fat and build muscle in the shortest time possible. It means that you change speeds while you exercise rather than always going full force or just plodding along. Exercising is more exciting that way, plus it gives you a chance to catch your breath after intense effort. What's not to like about that?

HERE ARE 10 SIMPLE INTERVAL WORKOUTS
THAT CAN GET YOU STARTED LOSING SERIOUS WEIGHT, WITHOUT
EVER FEELING EXHAUSTED OR BORED.

Hill repetitions

Find a decent-size hill. Begin by walking up it, then back down. Exertion going up, recovery coming back down. Simple, right? Do that for a couple of weeks, adding repetitions of going up and down as it gets easier, and soon you'll be ready to speedwalk or even jog up part of it. Continue that for a few more weeks, and you'll soon find that you can run or speedwalk all the way up before walking back down. There: You're an interval exerciser!

The telephone-pole game

You can do this one whether you're a walker, a runner, or a bicycler. When you start out, pick a geographical feature you'll see plenty of during your exercise—telephone poles work well, as do fire hydrants, mailboxes, etc.—and alternate speeding up and slowing down each time you see one.

Practically any team sport

If you're up to it, soccer, basketball, bowling, touch football, hockey, ultimate Frisbee, and even cartless golf (swing; walk; swing; walk some more; swing, swing, swing, curse, fling club, walk to retrieve club) will vary your exertion level and give you the interval benefit.

Office intervals

We already know about the slowed-down part: any time you're sitting at your desk. But you really need to be crafty about finding ways to escape your chair and stride through the workplace. You just need to change your mind-set. Instead of finding ways to remain rooted in place, look for reasons to stand up, move around, go for a walk, visit colleagues, and plot behind the boss's back. Bonus: Create a work area where you can stand up and spend part of the day working *and* standing. We'll call them standing intervals.

TV intervals

During all of the commercial breaks in primetime, commit to standing, or doing simple dumbbell curls, or circling the house once, or dropping for a set of pushups if you're inclined that way. You'll get in 20 minutes of workouts during the time you'd otherwise be watching commercials for the foods and restaurants that are making you fat. Activity is the best revenge.

Mall intervals

Park far from the entrance and commit to visiting at least a dozen stores and shopping for at least an hour. If you become overburdened with purchases, walk them back to the car, then resume shopping. It's a workout for your credit card, yes, but also for your cardiovascular

system. Walk right past the temptation of the soda and pretzel stands and pop a handful of the nuts you brought along.

Picnic intervals

And I do mean out—like, outdoors. Every region of the country has spectacular state parks that are underutilized as we nestle in for TV dinners that are making us fat. Distracted eaters consume up to 400 extra calories per chow session. Let's solve that problem by packing up food and finding wonderful places to eat it, like down the 1-mile trail to the river, the picnic table by the lake, or the top of the cliff overlooking the valley. You'll exercise on your way to dinner, you'll eat foods you prepared yourself, and you'll focus on what you're eating— three great new weight-loss advantages.

Volunteer intervals

Community service is an exercise program. During the park cleanup, you're engaging in varied activities while mingling with the right sorts of people—ones who care about your community. Join in with their most active programs, and they will crowd out

unproductive time you might lose to sedentary activities.

Water workouts

Canoeing. Kayaking. Row-row-rowing your boat gently down the stream. All of these self-propelled water sports require varied amounts of effort, and they also give you a new viewpoint. Off-road is the place where you engage your muscles and burn calories, and also gain new perspectives that are only available by leaving the blacktop.

In fact, any self-propelled activity

If you can just find ways to step out from behind the wheel or stand up from the chair, the world instantly changes. You're relying on your own muscular and energy systems to propel you through the landscape, and the view changes. You're self-reliant, you can move at your own preferred speed, and you can vary it to lend an extra calorie burn to things you're doing for enjoyment. Motorized machines don't love us; in fact, they're doing us in. Declare your independence and life will change for the better.

10
SECOND
SLIMDOWN

More Fun!

Some fitness tips are literally no-sweat—if you can build them into otherwise empty times of the day. And who doesn't have 10 seconds to try a new workout?

GET OUT OF THE CHAIR

Research has shown that obese people remain seated an average of 2 hours longer every day than skinny people. By remaining seated, they use 358 fewer calories every day, 2,506 fewer every week, and 130, 670 every year. (Mystery of obesity: solved!) Gives new meaning to the phrase "sentenced to the chair," doesn't it?

REPEAT AFTER US:

"Hey boy, want to go for a walk?" If you walk your dog for 15 minutes, you'll burn 61 calories. Do it three times a day: 183. Every day of the year: 467,565. And that's a very big deal: A new study from George Washington University shows that people who walk their dogs are half as likely to be overweight as couch-potato dog owners.

GO FOR THE CHOCOLATE MILK MOUSTACHE

A study from the University of Washington found that drinks that blend carbohydrates and protein— chocolate milk among them—do a 40 percent better job of helping your muscles recover and grow after a workout.

LIFT YOURSELF UP

Exercises like squats and pushups build metabolism-revving muscle in minutes and work just as well as fancy gym machines. If you tire your muscles in 60 to 90 seconds, your engine will be roaring.

FIRE THE MAID

Researchers reporting in the journal *Medicine and Science in Sports and Exercise* discovered that performing household chores reduces blood pressure. The scientists asked 28 people to do 150 calories' worth of housework daily. After 2 days, their BP levels fell an average of 13 points. And while the reductions lasted only 8 hours, daily chores could lower BP long-term, says lead author Jaume Padilla, M.S. Ask your spouse to help out more around the house—but only if he or she wants to live longer!

STAND UP WHEN YOU TALK ON THE PHONE

You won't think of it as exercise, but it can help you burn as much as 2.7 calories for every minute you're on the phone, and will subtly tone muscles that will serve you in a more active life. Bonus: Do a toe raise (exercise-speak for standing on your tiptoes) every time the conversation annoys you.

TAKE THE STAIRS

—rather than riding the elevator—for 2 or 3 minutes every day burns enough calories to halt the average American's weight gain of 1 to 2 pounds every year.

TARGET BELLY FAT

People who diet and exercise shrink their abdominal fat cells twice as much as those who diet only. Scientists studied people who had dropped an average of 22 pounds and observed that those who included exercise in their weight-loss programs were able to specifically target belly fat.

WALK 30 MINUTES EVERY DAY

It will burn about 120 calories, or a third of what you need to burn to lose 1 pound a week. A 10-minute walk after every meal will do it.

Lose Weight, 24/7

The gym isn't the answer to all your weight problems. Unless you lived there and worked out 8 hours a day, how could it be? Instead, start looking for opportunities to add movement, activity, and fun throughout your day. Channel flipping? Unfun. Romping with kids (and spouse)? Fun! Car commuting? Unfun. Biking to the farmer's market? Fun! Get the idea?

LEAN BELLY ACTIVITY PRESCRIPTION

REMEMBER HOW IT FELT TO GET THAT BICYCLE FOR YOUR 11TH BIRTHDAY? YOU CAN TAP THAT SPIRIT, AGAIN.

The Lean Living Turbocharge plan in Chapter 6 gave you four easy ways to add calorie-burning activity to your life.

→ **FOR EVERY HOUR YOU WATCH TV, COMMIT TO 15 MINUTES OF ACTIVITY.** Earn downtime with up-and-around time.

→ **ENGAGE YOUR SPOUSE, FAMILY, FRIENDS IN "PLAY" TIME.** Kids play, and so should you. Enlist "playmates," schedule fun activities, and make sure you follow through.

→ **SPEED UP, AND SLOW DOWN, TO LOSE WEIGHT.** Commit to three times a week for 20 minutes and exercise at a pace that varies from "kick it up" to "kicking back."

→ **TAKE ADVANTAGE OF NEAT.** Non-exercise activity thermogenesis is your best shot at burning significantly more calories without even noticing.

To put it all together, just turn the page. You'll soon have more fun, and fitness, in your life.

THE PERFECT WEEKDAY, WEEKNIGHT, SEASON, AND YEAR OF ACTIVITY

BURN MORE CALORIES AND WATCH YOUR ENERGY LEVELS SURGE BY FOLLOWING THE PRINCIPLES OF NEAT.

Non-exercise activity thermogenesis is simply a fancy way of saying that you don't have to pull on running shoes and sweats to work your body in ways that can help you live lighter, live more fully, live more enjoyably. Depending on how you use your time, your NEAT energy expenditure can vary by as much as 2,000 calories a day. Because you need to shed about 500 calories a day to lose 1 pound a week—by subtracting food from the diet, increasing activity, or both—NEAT is a great place to start. Here are some ways to do it.

Weekdays

Break the spell of the sedentary office.

• Park the car at the far side of the lot and hoof it to the building.

• Take a walk with co-workers for half the lunch hour.

• Once an hour, visit a co-worker rather than using the telephone or sending an e-mail.

• Stand during phone calls.

Weeknights

Reclaim your life from the screen.

• You already know what the TV is giving you: not much. Send the dog out to the backyard to bury the remote. Try something else. Take a 15-minute walk after dinner, or do physical household chores during the (many) dead spots in the TV schedule.

• Pursue a hobby that does not in any way involve a screen. Some examples: playing a musical instrument, woodworking, taking a classroom-based foreign-language course, volunteering at Meals on Wheels.

• One or two nights a week, go to a dance class or a basketball or bowling league game, tee off with a summer twilight golf league, or even take a stroll through the biggest mall in your area.

Weekends

You have the time, so move a muscle.

• Do a major home project that requires several hours of (enjoyable) physical labor, such as gardening, building, painting, or fixing. Bonus points if it requires mental labor to learn a new skill.

• Volunteer to coach youth sports teams, clean up the community, or help out with the church fair.

• Encounter nature for half a day: hike, walk, ride your bike along the local rail-to-trail route, explore your community on foot, canoe, kayak, golf (no cart!), go beachcombing, or go birding.

Once per season

Reach for a bigger goal.

• Escape on a weekend getaway that includes exploration by foot, bicycle, skis, running shoes, or boat.

• Participate in a charity walk, bike ride, or run.

Twice a year

Do something you can look forward to (and get in shape for).

• Take an active long-weekend-away with friends to camp, bike from one B&B to another, visit a national park or national seashore, or go hunting or fishing.

Once a year

Spend a big chunk of time outdoors to best bust stress.

• Immerse yourself in nature for a solid week. No, you don't have to sleep in a tent, but get outside every day for the same number of hours you'd put in inside on a workday. Get out on your feet, under the sky, and away from the electronic amusements and distractions that absorb far too much of our time. Clear your mind, fill your lungs with fresh air, and breathe out the stresses of our too-harried world.

• If you do all that, I guarantee you that a) this will be one of your most memorable years, b) you'll strengthen all of the relationships that matter most to you, plus make some new friendships, and c) you'll shed some of the heavy burden of inactivity. I'm not asking you to learn new exercises or sweat a bucketful. I'm merely asking you to pursue an active life and reap the rewards.

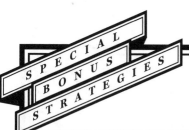
WEEK

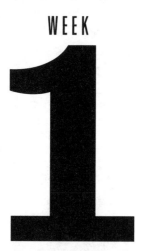

1

the PRESCRIPTION ACTIVITY PLANNER

Monday

Spend at least 30 minutes outside being active. Take a walk or bike ride after dinner, or stroll with workmates for half of your lunch hour.

Tuesday

Register for an active class.
After work today, or whenever you have a spare hour (there's a gap in the prime-time TV schedule, I assure you), find an active class you can sign up for in your community. It could be a dance class, a weekly yoga session, a hiking club, or a "biking for beginners" course. Now sign up, and commit to attending the classes every week for as long as they run.

Wednesday

Spend at least 30 minutes outside being active. Take a walk or bike ride after dinner, or stroll with workmates for half of your lunch hour.

Thursday

Today, start experimenting with NEAT: non-exercise activity thermogenesis. How? It's simple: Research shows that the more you sit, the greater your risk of heart disease, so stand when you're on the phone and walk instead of sending e-mails. Make it a point to look for opportunities to add activity to your day, and you can burn 1,000 extra calories this week.

Friday

Spend at least 30 minutes outside being active. Take a walk or bike ride after dinner, or stroll with work mates for half of your lunch hour.

Saturday

Play with kids for at least an hour. It's most convenient, obviously, if you have your own kids handy. Grandkids will also do, of course. Or borrow the neighbors'. Or find a community soccer league or youth sports league or church program where you can help out. Just find kids you can have fun with, and absorb their approach to activity: the sheer pleasure of movement. If there really aren't any kids around for you to play with, do this: play a game. If you once had an awesome jump shot, take a basketball to the park and shoot for half an hour. If you used to bike for miles as a kid, pull that bike out of the attic, dust it off, blow up the tires, and take an excursion around the block. Go bowling, walk the beach, or fly a kite. I'll even give you credit for mini-golf! Just remind yourself that physical activity is fun and sociable, and restore it to your regular list of pastimes as you bump aside sedentary fat-builders like TV watching and Web surfing.

Sunday

Experiment with intervals. As you learned on page 146, intervals are the best way to gain fitness and shed flab. But don't be intimidated by the name. "Doing intervals" simply means you'll be varying the speed at which you exercise. So if you're a walker, alternate 3 minutes of walking at a normal pace with 1 minute of fast walking. If you prefer bicycling, choose a route that will alternate between flat terrain and gentle hills. If you like to run, alternate your regular steady pace with short sprints. Remember, if you change the pace, you'll change your waist size.

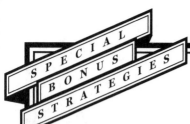

WEEK

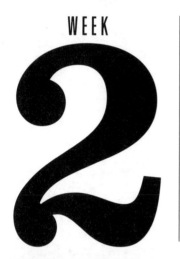

the PRESCRIPTION ACTIVITY PLANNER

Monday

Take a moment with your calendar to block out exercise time for the next 3 weeks. When I say "exercise," I mean half an hour of activity—walking, jogging, any of the simple workouts in Chapter 7—that you will promise yourself to engage in on 3 weekdays, starting today, with a longer session on Saturday or Sunday. (If you're a walker, take a hike on the weekend. Ride a bike? Drive to the country and do an extended tour. Shoot to double the amount of time you're exercising on workdays.) So I'm asking you to book 12 exercise sessions between now and the end of the month. When people try to schedule time with you, you can work around it. Or better yet, invite them to exercise with you, and book that date as well. **After dinner, take a walk of any length you choose.**

Tuesday

Participate in your activity class. It could be any day of the week, of course, just make sure you're signed up and ready to go.

Make it a NEAT day at the office, where you stand during phone calls, take the stairway instead of elevators, park farther from your building, walk to colleagues' offices instead of e-mailing, and generally look for ways to inject more activity into your daily routine.

Wednesday

30 minutes of activity.

Head out to a local sporting goods store and buy a pedometer. Play around with it this week, because it'll be a key part of your plan next week and going forward.

Thursday

After dinner, take a walk of any length you choose. Remember that NEAT can enliven your evening hours as well. Take your cues from the prime-time schedule: Whenever there's a commercial break in the action, lift light dumbbells for the duration of the commercials, vacuum the room at halftime (think how much your wife will appreciate it, guys!), or stand on your toes while you're waiting for the show to start again. There's a great list of NEAT exercises on page 152; pick some, and do them tonight!

Friday

30 minutes of activity.

Saturday

Plan a day outside with family and friends, whether it's renting canoes for a paddle on a nearby lake followed by a picnic, taking a hike in a nearby state park followed by a barbecue, or cross-country skiing and hot cocoa. The idea here: Make activity a prime entertainment option and motivation to get moving. Walking and jogging are not, in fact, the most exciting pursuits on the planet, but if they allow you to resume your downhill skiing hobby, or entice you to enter the 5-K charity run, or they pave the way for a vacation hike to the floor of the Grand Canyon, they can be steps toward the most fun you'll have in your life. Bonus: If you include friends and family in your preparation, they'll be with you for the adventures as well.

After dinner, take a walk of any length you choose with a friend or family member and talk about where your increased activity might take you in life. Brainstorm great plans, and build your fitness to realize them.

Sunday

Try an extended exercise session. Before kickoff, before you cook Sunday dinner, get in an exercise session that wouldn't be possible during the workweek. The goal here isn't to make you red-faced and panting, but to give you a sense of what it feels like to build your fitness levels and push yourself a little further and faster. As you do that, you'll find a new level of confidence and a new initiative to try activities that you might have thought were beyond you. Guess what, they're not!

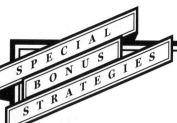
WEEK

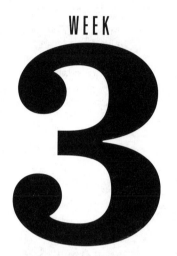
3

the PRESCRIPTION ACTIVITY PLANNER

Monday

I sent you out for a pedometer last Wednesday. So by now you know how to use it, right? I want you to wear it every day this week, and count up your total number of footsteps. If you've been experimenting with NEAT, now you'll have a chance to see what kinds of dividends it's paying. A British study showed that people who pay attention to the number of footsteps they take routinely add about 16 percent more activity to their days. That's why I love NEAT: It helps you insert calorie-burning motion into otherwise inactive spots in your days. And I know from personal experience that the more you're out and about, the more you're interacting with people, and the more you're seizing life's opportunities, the more energy you have. You don't exercise just for exercise's sake. You do it to live more fully.
Wear your pedometer for your regularly scheduled half hour of exercise, and make those steps count!

Tuesday

Your regularly scheduled activity night. Stick with it; you're starting to make friends there now, I bet. When they ask about your pedometer, tell 'em

Dr. Travis prescribed it for you. How many steps did you take today?

Wednesday

Your scheduled exercise day. During the half hour, see if you can reach a ratio of two-thirds regular pace to one-third accelerated intervals. Your body just told your belly: I'm going to burn you off.

How many steps today? Add a walk after dinner, just for bragging rights.

Thursday

Your day of NEAT. See if you can add 500 steps to the total you hit on Monday. Instead of driving to the strip mall for lunch, why don't you walk there and back? Have your sandwich at your desk, and your boss will never know you were out exercising.

Friday

Your scheduled exercise day. Now that we're in week 3, and you see how simple and pleasurable it is to add action to your life (and if it isn't, try different activities—this is about fun, not drudgery), take a look at the exercise programs in Chapter 7. Find one you think you could try, and schedule it for your extended exercise tomorrow. But read up on it now, practice the motions, and plan it out. You can buy any needed equipment tomorrow morning.

Saturday

Your weights workout. Try one of the muscle-building workouts from Chapter 7. There's also a good one in the bonus chapter starting on page 200. Many of these workouts call for light dumbbells, so start with 2 to 5 pounds. Other words for light dumbbells: a can of soup, even a small rock. Just pick something you can handle easily, and as you pile up the repetitions, you'll move on to heavier weights. But don't worry about that now. This is about being comfortable with weights, and the motions you make with them. Why bother? As you grow stronger, you'll tap into the 24-hour fat burn that muscle—and only muscle—can provide.

Sunday

Another day of active fun with people you love. This is my favorite part of *The Lean Belly Prescription*, and my ultimate goal for you: more energy to spend more time with people you love—this weekend, this lifetime.

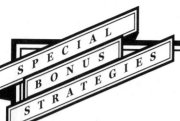
WEEK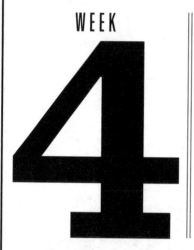

the PRESCRIPTION ACTIVITY PLANNER

Monday

This is the week you put it all together: You're wearing your pedometer, counting footsteps, and trying to boost your totals from one day to the next. You're aware of NEAT at home and in the office, to add activity and mobility to everything you do. You've got your class on Tuesday night, and you're making plans for a full day of fun on Sunday. On Saturday, you'll have an extended exercise session, to introduce some sweat

to leisure time. And for all of that, you've essentially added only a few more than 2 hours to your weekly schedule for exercise, while packing in more fun and sociality in times when you might just have been staring at one screen or another. Do you see what's happened? You've gone from being a person defined by the imprint your bottom makes on various chairs, to one defined by your ability to interact with the people and world around you. This isn't

just exercise, it's a process of becoming a whole new you— with a whole lot less flesh and more fun!

Regularly scheduled exercise, and keep counting your footsteps.

Tuesday

Your regularly scheduled class, plus the NEAT advantage all day long.

Wednesday

Regularly scheduled exercise, plus a walk

after dinner. If you're a morning person, why not take one before breakfast, as well? You know the concept of sneaking a snack at the refrigerator? Why not find time to sneak in exercise, as well. Doing it for as little as 5 minutes here and there can have a positive impact on your fitness levels. If you keep track of the time, you can watch it build up. Five minutes more here, 5 minutes more there, and suddenly it's a pound less this week, 2 pounds less next. Celebrate the improvements in small increments, and soon you'll see big benefits over longer stretches of time.

Thursday

Beat last Thursday's footstep totals by another 500. The more you add, the more inches you subtract from your waistline.

Friday

Your regularly scheduled exercise. You're gaining skill and confidence now, and your routine may begin feeling easier. Look for opportunities to increase the weight you're using—just a little, don't go crazy now!—or the pace at which you're exercising. You don't need to add hours, just intensity, to grow increasingly fit. That's the interval advantage: When your fast pace equals or betters your moderate pace, you'll maximize your fat-burning.

Saturday

You've got the time, so try another weight-lifting workout from Chapter 7. All of the exercise programs in this book are total-body workouts, so they'll help you build more muscle from head to toe, but also increase your agility and strength for sports. One of the best ways to make sure you get your workout in is to have friends who are looking forward to seeing you on the walking trail, on the court, on the bike path, or in the lift line. That's really why you're doing this: to increase the number of activities you enjoy and the number of friends and family members who will enjoy them with you. Losing weight is simply a side benefit—and a back and front benefit, too.

Sunday

Another day pursuing an activity you enjoy with people you love. Spend the day at it, enjoy the progress that you've made, and cook a meal that tastes good and is good for you. Now do the most important exercise of the whole bunch: Plan your next 4 weeks of food, fun, and activity. You're already miles beyond where you were 1 month ago, but not as far ahead as you'll be at the end of the month. That's the best thing about my prescription: It can last a lifetime, and will yield benefits every step of the way.

Next month? Why, your best ever, of course!

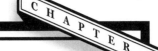

CHAPTER 7

The World's Easiest Exercise Plan

Turbocharge **The Lean Belly Prescription**
with any one of these fat-blasting,
muscle-making fitness plans.

〜〜〜〜〜〜〜〜〜〜〜〜〜〜〜〜〜〜〜〜〜〜〜

I've already noted that the best way to add activity to your life is to do it when you're not formally exercising. Look at it this way: Your most annoying workout-freak friends are only spending

5 percent of their waking hours doing formal exercise plans. That's 5 hours a week. The key for all the rest of us is to burn more fat during the other 95 percent of the week. Any of the no-excuse fitness plans I outlined in Chapter 6 will help you do that. But even as you're upping the activity you build into everyday life, you should consider adding a formal workout as well. It will help build lean muscle—a major fat incinerator—and add healthy structure to your week. (And don't worry about "bulking up." You'd need to spend *a lot* of time lifting *a lot* of weight before that could happen!) It needn't be intimidating. You can do most of these workouts while watching the tube or listening to tunes. And you can do them with your spouse, best friend, or kids.

So try these workouts, and see which suits you and your friends and family. No suffering allowed! "Fun" is the new "fit," after all.

CHAPTER

7

LAWS OF

LEANNESS

You can get fit and burn calories all day, even when you're not "exercising."

To lose maximum weight, exercise your biggest muscles: chest, butt, back, abs, and legs.

Almost any exercise can be done at home with a pair of light dumbbells.

Muscle is a metabolic inferno; it burns fat for hours after you're done exercising.

A day of rest after each workout is critical to allow your muscles to recover.

The best program is one that gets tougher as you get tougher!

THE RIGHT WORKOUT FOR EVERY BODY

How do we know this workout will work for you? Because there are three variations—beginner, intermediate, expert—that you can use according to your current fitness level. Whether you've never worked out before or have been hitting the gym for years, there's a cutting-edge, fat-blasting routine that's right for your body.

Choose Your Lean-Belly Workout Plan

The Special Bonus Strategies following this chapter has additional workout options. Whichever workout you choose, it's designed to elevate your heart rate, get you breathing hard, and work every muscle in your body. The upshot: You'll burn fat fast while boosting your fitness to an all-time high. For each of these exercises, use a weight you can lift comfortably for the recommended number of repetitions while maintaining proper form.

OPTION 1 *The Beginner Workout* Choose this plan if you're more than 25 pounds overweight, or if you haven't consistently been doing resistance training 3 days a week for the past 3 months.

OPTION 2 *The Intermediate Workout* Choose this plan if you've regulaly lifted weights for the past 3 months, but have less than 6 months' experience.

OPTION 3 *The Expert Workout* Choose this plan if you've been lifting weights at least 3 days a week for 6 months or more.

How to Do the Workouts

Once you choose your workout plan, you're ready to get started. You'll see that each plan has two routines: Workout A and Workout B. Simply alternate between these two workouts 3 days a week, resting a day between each session. So in week 1, you might do Workout A on Monday and Friday, and Workout B on Wednesday. In week 2, you'd then do Workout B on Monday and Friday, and Workout A on Wednesday.

Perform the workouts as a circuit, completing the prescribed number of repetitions for each. That is, do one exercise after another, resting as little as possible between each. So you'll do one set of exercise 1, one set of exercise 2, then one set of exercise 3, and so on, until you've completed one set of all five exercises. Then rest long enough to catch your breath. That's one circuit. Use the guide below to tailor the workout to your fitness level.

BEGINNER: Do 2 to 3 circuits.
If needed, rest for up to 30 seconds between each exercise. Try to rest a little less each time you do the workout.

INTERMEDIATE: Do 3 circuits.

EXPERT: Do 3 to 4 circuits.

Simple, right? Now let's get started.

WORKOUT

A

BEGINNER

1 *Beginner Plank*

Assume a pushup position, but with your elbows bent and forearms resting on a bench. Your body should form a straight line. Now tighten your core by making your stomach as skinny as you can, and hold that position for 30 seconds. (If that's too hard, hold for 5 seconds, relax, and hold again.)

Hold for 30 seconds

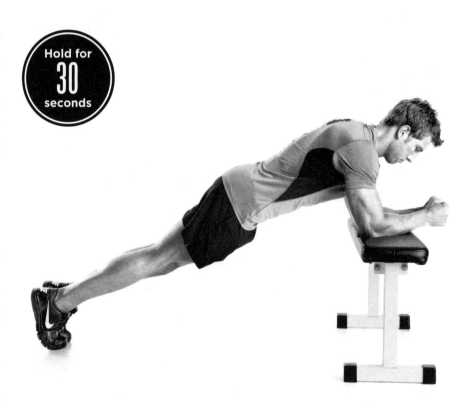

WORKOUT

A

BEGINNER

2 *Dumbbell Stepup*

Grab a pair of light dumbbells, and place your left foot on a step that's about knee-height. Press your left heel into the step and push your body up until your left leg is straight. (Don't rest your right foot on the step.) Lower back down and repeat. Do all your reps; then switch legs. If that's too hard, use a lower step.

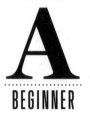

Do
8 to **10**
repetitions
(each leg)

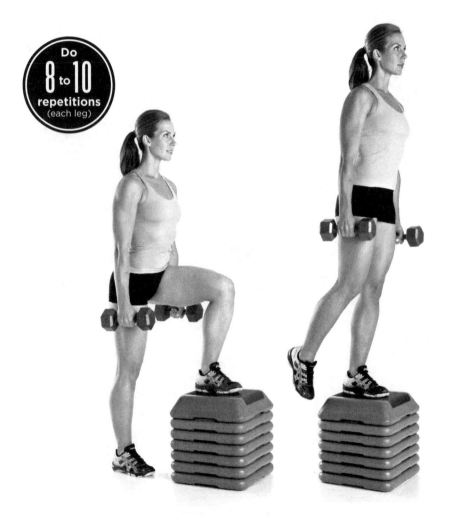

WORKOUT

A

BEGINNER

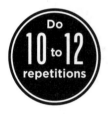

3 *Bent-Over T*

Grab a pair of dumbbells, bend at your hips and knees (don't round your lower back), and lower your torso until it's nearly parallel to the floor. Let your arms hang straight down from your shoulders, your palms facing forward. Now raise your arms straight out to your sides until they're in line with your body. Lower and repeat.

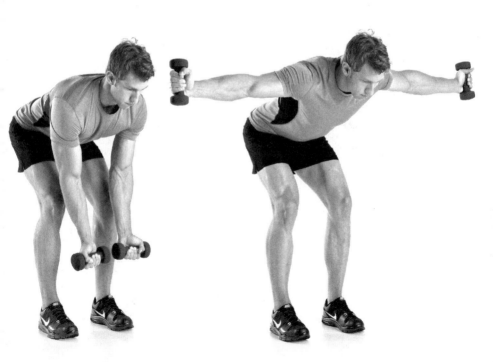

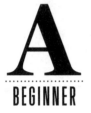

WORKOUT

A

BEGINNER

4 *Body-Weight Squat*

Stand as tall as you can with your feet set slightly wider than shoulder-width apart. Hold your arms straight out in front of your body at shoulder level. Keeping your lower back naturally arched, slowly lower your body as far as you can by pushing your hips back and bending your knees. Pause, then push yourself back to the start.

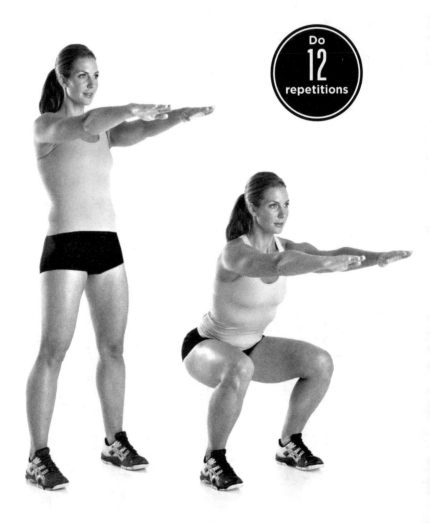

Do
12
repetitions

WORKOUT

A

BEGINNER

5 *Beginner Pushup*

Assume a pushup position, only place your hands on a raised surface—such as a bench or step—instead of the floor. Then bend your elbows and lower your body until your chest nearly touches the raised surface. Pause, and then push yourself back to the start. If that's too hard, use an even higher surface so that you're more upright.

Do
10 to 15
repetitions

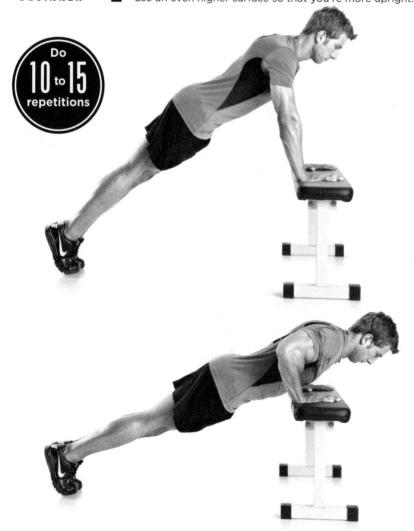

B

BEGINNER

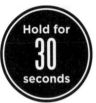

Hold for
30
seconds

1 *Beginner Side Plank*

Place your left forearm on a bench, and turn your body so that you're facing sideways (as shown). Raise your hips so that your body forms a straight line. Now tighten your core by making your stomach as skinny as you can, and hold for 30 seconds. If that's too hard, just hold as long as you can. Then repeat for your other side.

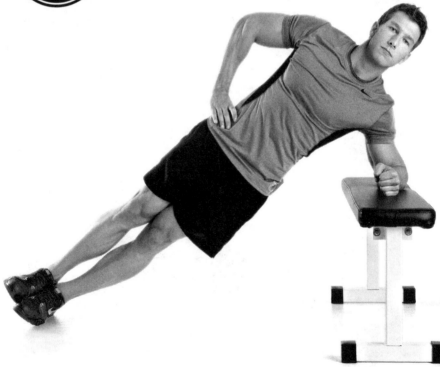

2 *Dumbbell Split Squat*

Hold a pair of dumbbells at arm's length next to your sides, your palms facing each other. Stand in a staggered stance with your left foot in front of your right. Slowly lower your body as far as you can. Pause, then push yourself back up to the starting position. Do all your reps, then switch foot positions and repeat.

Do
8 to 10
repetitions

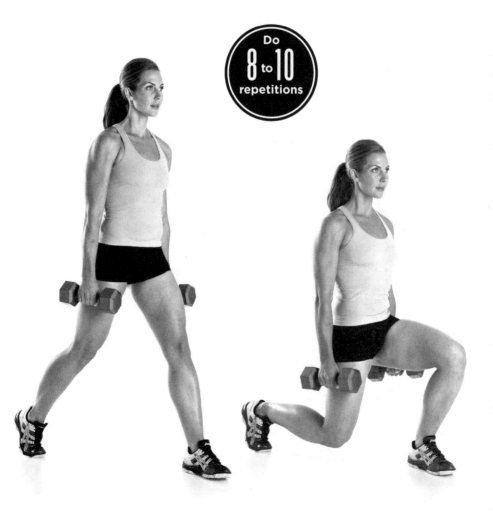

WORKOUT

B

BEGINNER

3 Dumbbell Row

Grab a pair of dumbbells, bend at your hips (don't round your lower back), and lower your torso until it's nearly parallel to the floor. Let the dumbbells hang at arm's length. Without moving your torso, squeeze your shoulder blades together and pull the weights to the sides of your torso. Pause, then lower back to the start.

Do 8 to 10 repetitions

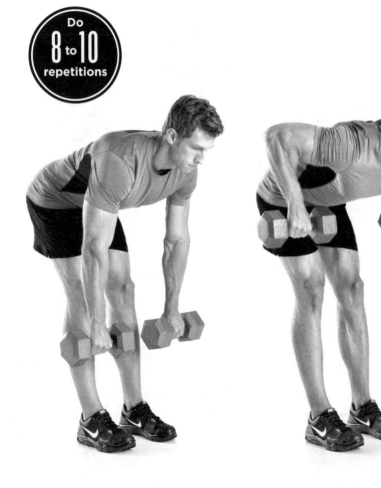

WORKOUT

B

BEGINNER

4 *Hip Raise*

Lie on your back with your knees bent and your feet flat. Tighten your core (as you do for the plank and side plank), squeeze your buttocks (glutes), and lift your hips until your body forms a straight line from knees to shoulders. Hold for 5 seconds—keep squeezing your glutes tightly—and return to the starting position. That's 1 rep.

Do **10** to **12** repetitions

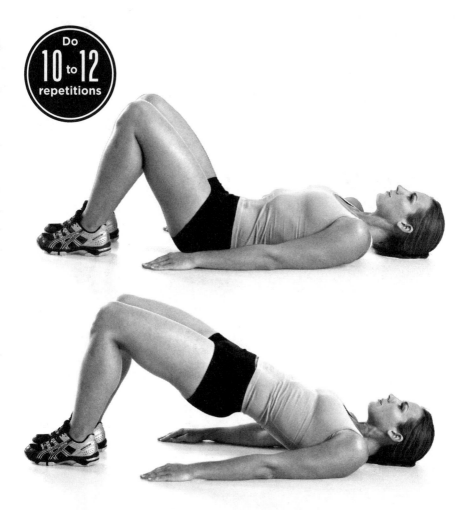

WORKOUT

B

BEGINNER

5 *Standing T and Shrug*

Stand holding a pair of dumbbells at arm's length next to your sides, your palms facing each other. Without changing the bend in your elbows, raise your arms at an angle to your body (so that they form a horizontal "Y") until they're at shoulder level. At the top of the move, shrug your shoulders upward. Pause, lower, and repeat.

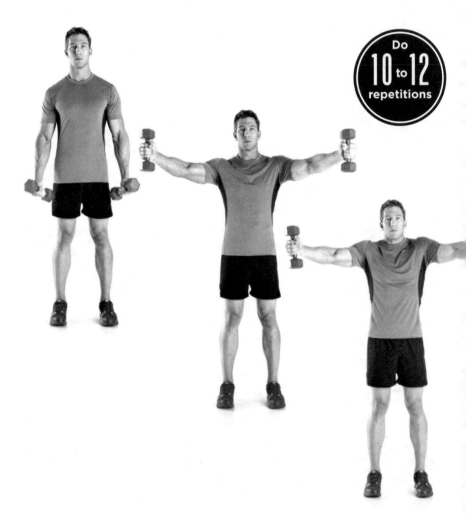

Do **10** to **12** repetitions

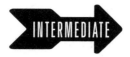

INTERMEDIATE

WORKOUT

A

INTERMEDIATE

1 *Plank*

Assume a pushup position, but with your elbows bent and forearms resting on the floor. Your body should form a straight line. Now tighten your core by making your stomach as skinny as you can, and hold that position for 30 seconds. If that's too hard, use the beginner plank from the Beginner Workout.

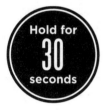

Hold for
30
seconds

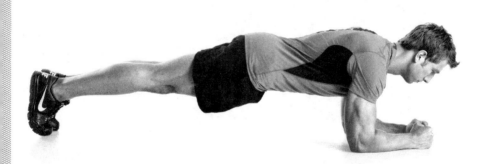

WORKOUT

A
INTERMEDIATE

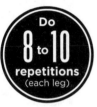

Do
8 to 10
repetitions
(each leg)

2 *Dumbbell Crossover Stepup*

Grab a pair of dumbbells and stand with an 18" step to your right. Cross your left foot in front of your body and place it on the step. Press your left foot into the step and push your body up until your left leg is straight. Slowly lower yourself back down. Do all your reps, and then turn around and repeat with your right leg.

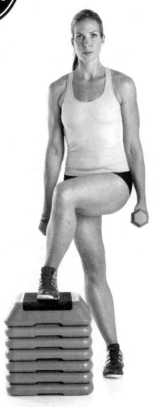

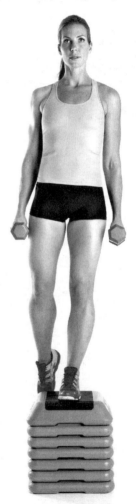

WORKOUT

A

INTERMEDIATE

3 *Bent-Over Y*

Grab a pair of dumbbells, bend at your hips and knees (don't round your lower back), and lower your torso until it's nearly parallel to the floor. Let your arms hang straight down from your shoulders. Now raise your arms at an angle to your body (so that they form a Y) until they're in line with your torso. Pause, lower, and repeat.

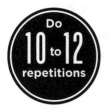

Do **10** to **12** repetitions

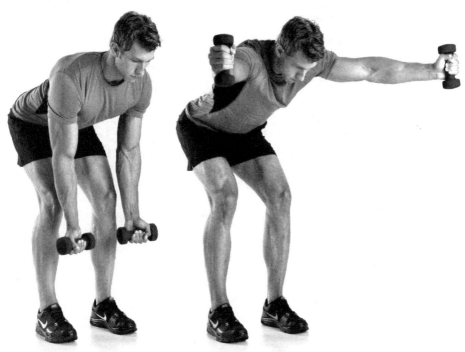

WORKOUT

A

INTERMEDIATE

4 *Goblet Squat*

With both hands, grab one end of a dumbbell to hold it vertically in front of your chest, and set your feet slightly beyond shoulder-width. Keeping your back naturally arched, push your hips back, bend your knees, and lower your body until the tops of your thighs are at least parallel to the floor. Pause, and push back up.

Do 12 repetitions

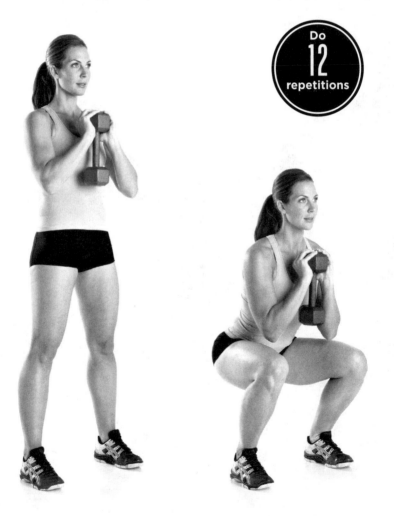

A

INTERMEDIATE

Do 10 to 12 repetitions

5 Pushup

Get down on all fours and place your hands on the floor so that they're slightly wider than your shoulders. Your body should form a straight line. Bend your elbows and lower your body until your chest nearly touches the floor. Pause, and then push yourself back to the start. If that's too hard, use the beginner pushup.

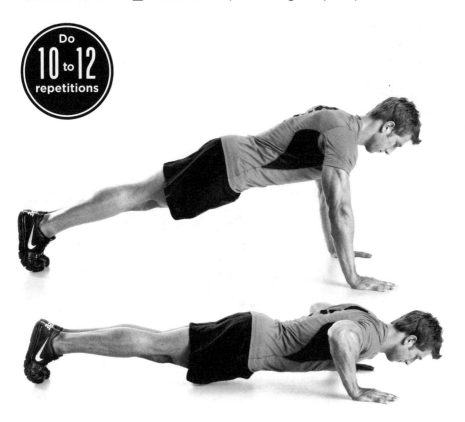

WORKOUT

B

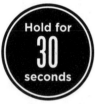

INTERMEDIATE

1 *Side Plank*

Lie on one side with your legs straight, and prop your upper body up on your forearm (as shown). Raise your hips so that your body forms a straight line. Now tighten your core by making your stomach as skinny as you can, and hold for 30 seconds. If that's too hard, do the beginner side plank. Then repeat for your other side.

Hold for 30 seconds

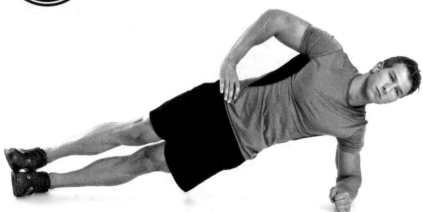

WORKOUT

B

INTERMEDIATE

2 *Offset Dumbbell Split Squat*

Hold a dumbbell at arm's length next to your right side. Stand in a staggered stance with your right foot in front of your left. Slowly lower your body as far as you can. Pause, then push yourself back up to the starting position. Do all your reps, then switch arms and legs, and repeat.

Do **8** to **10** repetitions

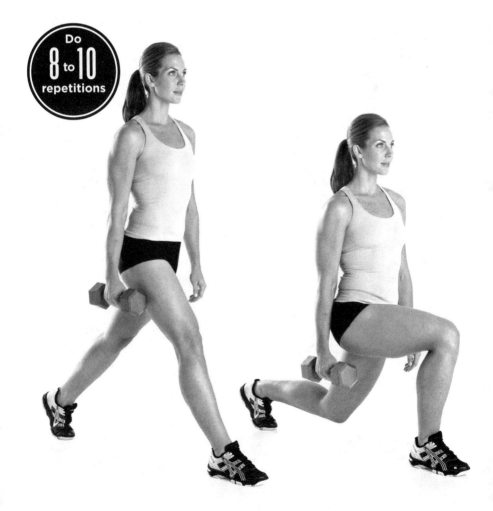

WORKOUT

B

INTERMEDIATE

Do 8 to 10 repetitions

3 *Alternating Dumbbell Row*

Grab a pair of dumbbells, bend at your hips (don't round your lower back), and lower your torso until it's nearly parallel to the floor. Let the dumbbells hang at arm's length. Without moving your torso, lift one dumbbell to your side, lower, and repeat with your other arm. That's 1 rep.

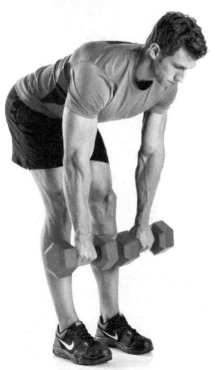
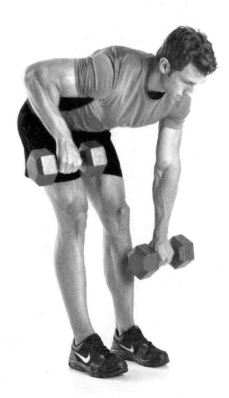

WORKOUT

B

INTERMEDIATE

4 *Dumbbell Straight-Leg Deadlift*

Grab a pair of dumbbells and hold them at arm's length in front of your thighs, palms facing your body. Your knees should be slightly bent and feet shoulder-width apart. Without rounding your lower back, bend at your hips and lower your torso until it's nearly parallel to the floor. Pause and then rise back to the starting position.

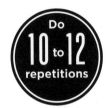

Do **10** to **12** repetitions

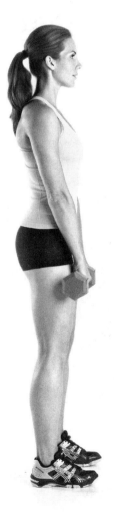

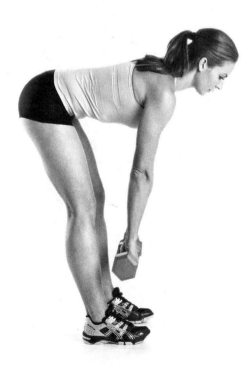

WORKOUT

B

INTERMEDIATE

5 *Dumbbell Shoulder Press*

Stand tall holding a pair of dumbbells just outside of your shoulders, with your arms bent and palms facing each other. Now press the weights directly over your shoulders until your arms are completely straight. Then slowly lower the dumbbells to the starting position.

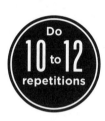

Do
10 to **12**
repetitions

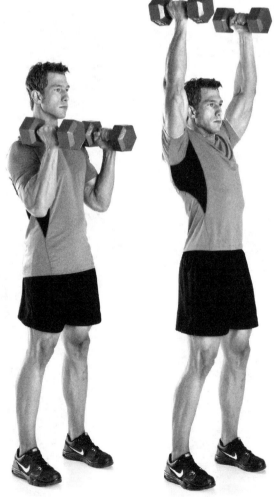

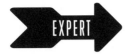
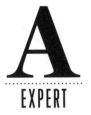

WORKOUT

A

EXPERT

1 *Plank with Feet on Bench*

Assume a pushup position, but with your elbows bent and forearms resting on the floor, and your feet placed on a bench (as shown). Your body should form a straight line. Now tighten your core by making your stomach as skinny as you can, and hold that position for 30 seconds. If that's too hard, do the intermediate or beginner plank instead.

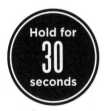

Hold for
30
seconds

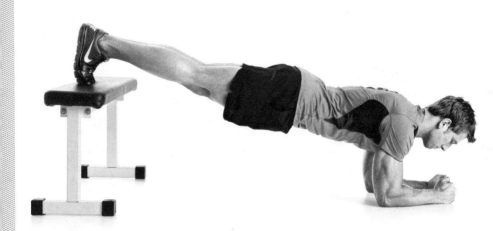

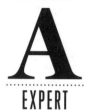

WORKOUT

A

EXPERT

2 *One-Leg Straight-Leg Deadlift*

Grab a pair of dumbbells and hold them at arm's length in front of your thighs, palms facing your body. Lift one foot off the floor. Without rounding your lower back, bend at your hips and lower your torso until it's nearly parallel to the floor. Pause and then rise back to the start. Do all your reps, then switch legs and repeat.

Do 8 to 10 repetitions (each leg)

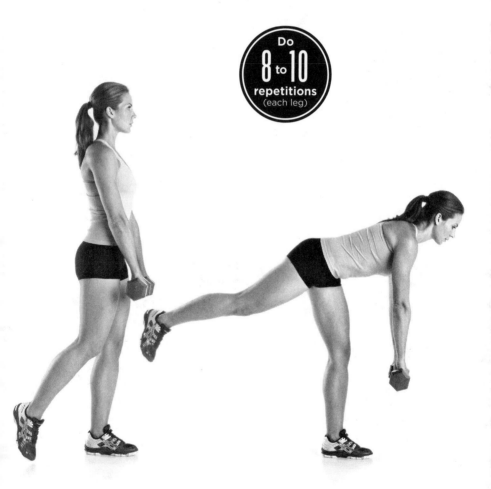

3 *Bent-Over L Raise*

Grab a pair of dumbbells, bend at your hips, and lower your torso (as shown). Let your arms hang down, palms facing your body. Keeping your upper arms perpendicular to your torso, bend your elbows and lift the weights. Then without changing your elbow position, rotate your forearms up. Pause, then reverse to the start.

Do
10 to **12**
repetitions

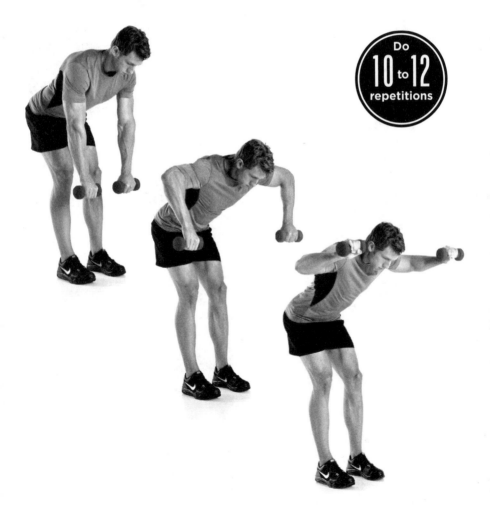

A

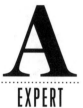

EXPERT

4 *Overhead Dumbbell Squat*

Stand holding a pair of dumbbells directly over your shoulders, your arms straight. Keeping your torso as upright as possible, push your hips back, bend your knees, and lower your body until your upper thighs are parallel to the floor. Don't let the dumbbells fall forward as you squat. Pause, then push back to the start.

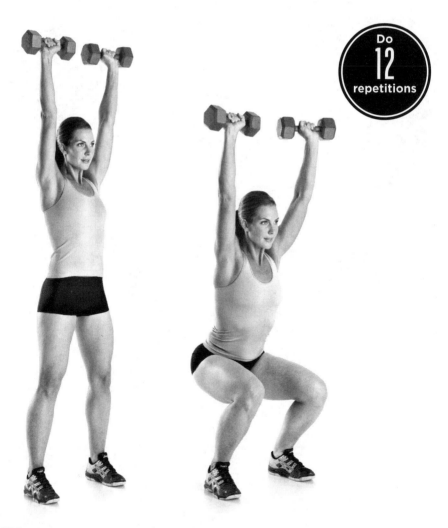

Do
12
repetitions

WORKOUT

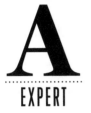

EXPERT

5 *T-Pushup*

Grab a pair of hex dumbbells and assume a pushup position. Bend your elbows and lower your body until your chest nearly touches the floor. As you push back up, lift your right hand, rotate the right side of your body, and raise the dumbbell straight up over your shoulder until your body forms a T. Repeat, this time rotating left.

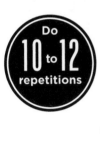

Do 10 to 12 repetitions

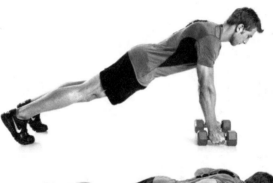

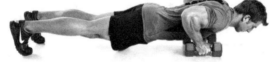

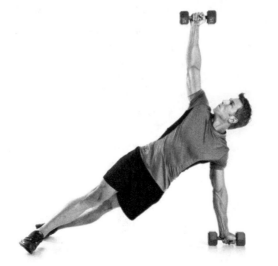

WORKOUT

B

·········

EXPERT

1 *One-Leg Side Plank*

Lie on one side with your legs straight, and prop your upper body up on your forearm. Raise your hips so that your body forms a straight line. Then raise your top leg (as shown) and hold it there. Now tighten your core by making your stomach as skinny as you can, and hold for 30 seconds. Repeat for your other side.

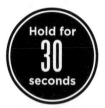

Hold for
30
seconds

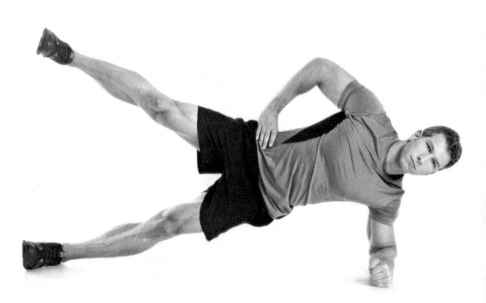

WORKOUT

B

EXPERT

2 *Overhead Split Squat*

Hold a pair of dumbbells directly over your shoulders, with your arms straight. Stand in a staggered stance with your left foot in front of your right. Slowly lower your body as far as you can. Pause, then push yourself back up to the start. Do all your reps, then switch legs and repeat.

Do 8 to 10 repetitions

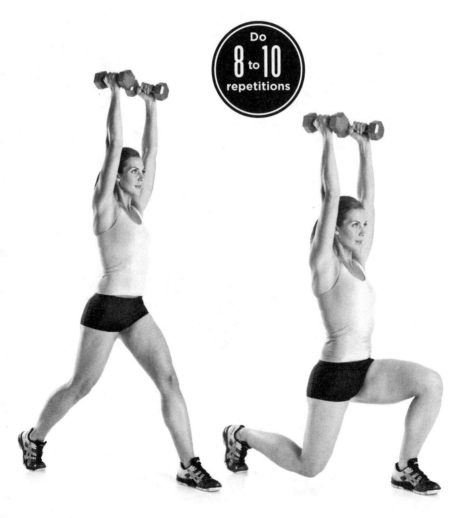

3 *One-Leg Neutral-Grip Row*

Grab a pair of dumbbells and balance on one leg. Bend at your hips and knees, and lower your torso until it's nearly parallel to the floor. Let the dumbbells hang at arm's length from your shoulders, palms facing each other. Without moving your torso, pull the weights to the sides of your torso. Pause, then lower to the start.

Do
8 to 10
repetitions

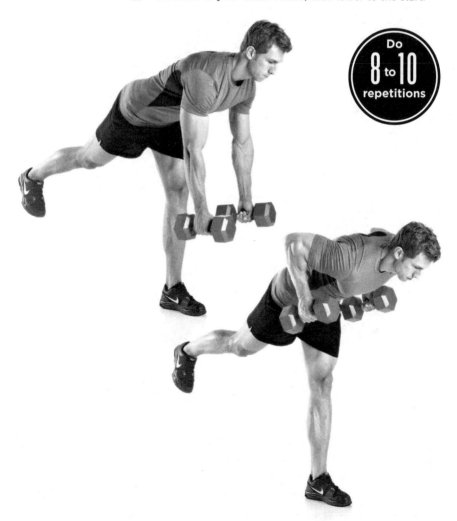

WORKOUT

B

EXPERT

Do
10 to 12
repetitions

4 *Dumbbell Swing*

Stand with your feet just beyond shoulder-width, your knees slightly bent. Hold a dumbbell with both hands at arm's length. To start, swing the weight back between your legs (don't round your lower back) and then thrust your hips forward and stand up, allowing momentum to swing the weight to shoulder height. That's 1 rep.

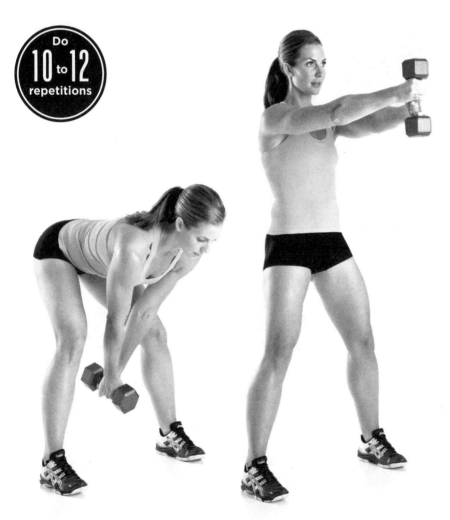

WORKOUT

B

EXPERT

5 *Alternating Shoulder Press*

Stand holding a pair of dumbbells just outside of your shoulders, with your arms bent and palms facing each other. Press the dumbbell in your left hand straight above your shoulder until your arm is straight. As you lower the weight, press the dumbbell in your right hand. That's 1 rep. Continue to alternate back and forth.

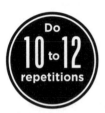

Do **10** to **12** repetitions

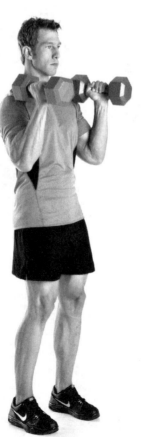

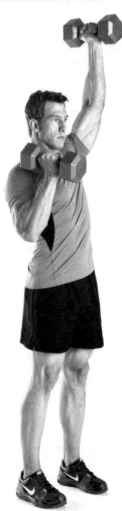

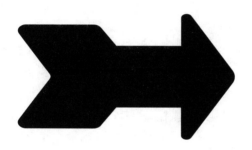

10 SECOND SLIMDOWN | More Muscle

Exercise isn't just something you do in the gym. All movement and activity counts, including things you actually enjoy doing!

LOSE FAT FASTER

Performing 8 to 15 repetitions per set works the best for fat loss. Research shows that performing sets in this range stimulates the greatest increase in fat-burning hormones, compared with doing a greater or fewer number of reps. Twelve to 15 reps is a great place to start, especially for beginners.

FIND YOUR IDEAL WEIGHT

Lift the heaviest weight that allows you to complete all of the prescribed repetitions. That is, the lower number of reps, the heavier the weight you should use. And vice versa. Remember, the goal is to complete all the reps in each set with perfect form.

CONTROL YOUR BLOOD SUGAR

Biceps offer more than flex appeal: Muscle reduces levels of insulin resistance, a red flag for diabetes, say UCLA scientists. Without enough muscle, your body struggles to use insulin to regulate blood sugar, which may trigger type 2 diabetes.

SHORTCUT TO 32" JEANS

Replacing flab with muscle will shrink your waist size. That's because 1 pound of fat takes up 18 percent more space on your body than 1 pound of muscle.

DOUBLE THE BENEFIT

Staying active provides a double dose of weight-loss fuel: On top of burning calories, exercise helps your brain stick to a healthy eating plan, according to University of Pittsburgh researchers. Exercise is a reminder to stay on track, reinforcing your weight-loss goal and drive.

DO IT LIKE POPEYE

A study at the Boston University Medical Center showed that people who consumed high levels of vitamin C were three times less likely to strain or injure joints than those who consumed the lowest levels. And vitamin E has been shown to reduce pain for people with arthritis. A great source of C and E: spinach, of course.

TAME A RAGING APPETITE

Contrary to popular belief, exercise doesn't spur you to eat more later in the day, say British researchers. In their study, men who ran on a treadmill for 90 minutes consumed just as many calories over the next 24 hours as they did on the days they didn't work out. The likely reason: Exercise may suppress appetite.

WATCH LESS, WEIGH LESS

Shed pounds with the press of a button. A recent Stanford University study found that people who cut their daily tube time by half (to 2.5 hours, on average) burned 120 calories more per day than those who continued to watch their usual amount. "Most increased their calorie burn through light activities like cleaning the house," says lead study author Jennifer Otten, Ph.D. This could help you lose 12 pounds or more in a year.

Workouts That Don't Feel Like Work

Changing your attitude toward exercise might just be as simple as changing the kinds of exercise you're doing. Here are some great ideas on how to work out anywhere, anytime, and have more fun doing it! Start here, slim there.

20 WAYS TO STICK TO YOUR WORKOUT

You have the right to remain fat. Or skinny. Or weak. But you should know that every workout you miss can and will be used against you to make your belly bigger, your muscles smaller and weaker, and your life shorter. Unfortunately, most Americans are exercising their right not to exercise.

A recent study by the National Center for Health Statistics found that only 19 percent of the population regularly engages in "high levels of physical activity." (That's defined as three intense 20-minute workouts per week.) Another 63 percent—about the same percentage as that of Americans who are overweight—believe that exercising would make them healthier, leaner, and less stressed, but they don't do it. At the root of this problem is motivation—or, rather, the lack thereof.

It's the difference between wanting to exercise and actually doing it. Follow the advice here, and rediscover the fun of fitness.

1 Sign up for a distant race. That is, one that's at least 500 miles away. The extra incentive of paying for airfare and a hotel room will add to your motivation to follow your training plan.

2 Make a "friendly" bet. Challenge your nemesis—that idea-stealing co-worker or nonmowing neighbor—to a contest. The first one to drop 15 pounds, run a 7-minute mile, or bench-press 150 pounds wins. (It's okay if your rival thinks you're best friends.)

3 Tie exercise to your health. Check your cholesterol. Then set a goal of lowering your LDL cholesterol by 20 points and increasing your HDL cholesterol by 5 points. Ask your doctor to write a prescription for new blood work in a month. You'll just have to go to the lab, and the doctor will call you with the results.

4 Switch your training partners.
Working out with a partner who will hold you accountable for showing up at the gym works well—for a while. But the more familiar you are with the partner, the easier it becomes to back out of workout plans. To keep this from happening, find a new, less forgiving workout partner every few months, if necessary.

5 Compete.
Find a sport or event that you enjoy, and train to compete in it. "It adds a greater meaning to each workout," says Alex Koch, Ph.D., C.S.C.S., an exercise researcher (and competitive weight lifter) at Truman State University in Kirksville, Missouri.

6 Think about fat.
Your body is always storing and burning fat, but at any given time it's doing more of one than the other. "Understanding that you're getting either fatter or leaner at any one time will keep you body conscious so you won't overeat or underexercise," says Alwyn Cosgrove, C.S.C.S., co-owner of Results Fitness in Santa Clarita, California.

7 Do a daily gut check.
Place your fingers on your belly and inhale deeply so it expands. As you exhale, contract your abdominal muscles and push your fingertips against your hard abdominal wall. Now pinch. "You're holding pure fat between your fingers," says Tom Seabourne, Ph.D., co-author of *Athletic Abs*. Do this every day, 30 minutes before your workout, and you'll find that you rarely decide to skip it.

8 Join a fitness or weight-loss message board.
It'll be full of inspiration from people who have accomplished their goals and are working toward new ones. We've started one at LeanBellyRx. com. Care to join?

9 Make an agreement with your spouse and kids.
The rule: You each get 1 hour to yourself every day, provided that you use it for exercise. So there's no pressure to do household chores, play marathon games of Monopoly, or be a doting spouse (a fat, doting spouse).

10 Burn a workout CD.

Studies have shown that people who pedal stationary cycles while listening to their favorite music will do so for longer and more intensely than those who exercise without music. So create a playlist with your favorite adrenaline-boosting songs.

11 Plan your workouts in advance.

At the start of each month, schedule all of your workouts at once, and cross them off as they're completed. For an average month, you might try for a total of 16 workouts. If any are left undone at the end of the month, tack them on to the following month. And make sure you have a contingency plan for bad weather and unscheduled meetings.

12 Squat first.

If you have trouble finishing your workout, start with the exercises you dread. "You'll look forward to your favorite exercises at the end of your workout, which will encourage you to complete the entire session," says John Williams, C.S.C.S., co-owner of Spectrum Conditioning Systems in Port Washington, New York.

13 Schedule a body-composition test every 2 months.

It'll provide you with a clear end date for the simple goal of losing body fat or gaining muscle. Your gym probably offers the service for a small fee—just make sure the same trainer performs the test each time.

14 Don't do what you hate.

"Whenever you start to dread your workout, do what appeals to you instead," says John Raglin, Ph.D., an exercise psychologist at Indiana University in Bloomington. If you despise the treadmill, then jump rope, lift weights, or hit a basketball court. Bottom line: If you're sick of your routine, find a new one.

15 Go through the motions.

On days when you don't feel like working out, make the only requirement of your exercise session a single set of your favorite exercise. "It's likely that once you've started, you'll finish," says Rachel Cosgrove, C.S.C.S. If you still don't feel like being active, go home. This way, you never actually stop exercising; you'll just have some gaps in your training log.

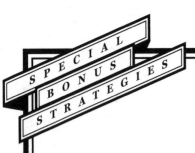
16 Start a streak. There's nothing like a winning streak to attract fans to the ballpark. Do the same for your workout by trying to set a new record for consecutive workouts without a miss. Every time your streak ends, strive to set a longer mark in your next attempt.

17 Make your goals attractive. "To stay motivated, frame your goals so that they drive you to achieve them," says Charles Staley, C.S.C.S., owner of Staley Training Systems. For some, running for charity works. For others, a body metric is motivating (losing 15 pounds, say). Others may want to schedule a vacation as a reward for a specific goal they've achieved. Whatever excites you most: Go for it!

18 See your body through his or her eyes. Ask your partner to make like Howard Stern and identify your most displeasing physical characteristic. It's instant motivation. If he or she is hesitant, make a list— abs, love handles, upper arms, and so on—and have him or her rank them from best to worst. Make the most-hated body part your workout focus for 4 weeks, then repeat the quiz for more motivation.

19 Join the best gym, not the best-priced one. If you lay out for a sweat shop with the best facilities, location, and clientele, it'll cost you. But you'll be motivated to attend for two reasons: It's a cool place to be, and also because you won't want to waste the good money you're spending on it. Plus there will be a certain amount of social pressure to make progress, with all of those fit bodies around.

20 Ramp up the pressure. Schedule a beach vacation. RSVP to the high school reunion. Challenge your best friends to a competition. Set a deadline, complete with dire consequences if you fail. Tell all your friends your goals, along with a specific date when you plan to achieve them. Whatever it takes to drive your performance going forward, do it.

EXERCISE ANYWHERE, ANYTIME!

TRAVELING? NO EQUIPMENT? NO GYM? TRY THIS SIMPLE,
WHOLE-BODY PLAN FROM ALWYN COSGROVE, C.S.C.S.,
CO-OWNER OF RESULTS FITNESS IN SANTA CLARITA, CALIFORNIA.

Do 10 reps of this exercise. (One second up, 1 second down, and a 1-second pause in between. That'll take 30 seconds. Then rest 1 minute.)

Repeat this process, moving to a new exercise every minute, until you've completed all five exercises. That's 1 circuit. Do a total of 4 circuits.

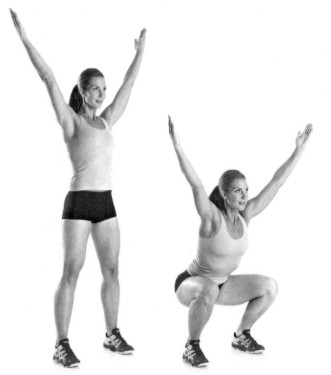

EXERCISE 1 *Y Squat*

Stand and raise your arms so your body forms a Y. Pull your shoulder blades together, and squat as deeply as you can by pushing your hips back and bending your knees. Then push back up.

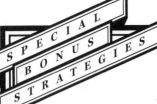
EXERCISE ANYWHERE, ANYTIME!

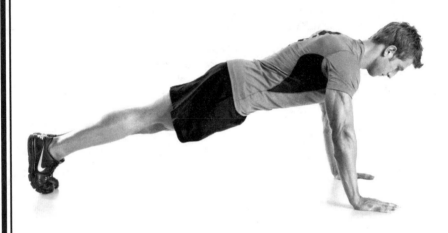

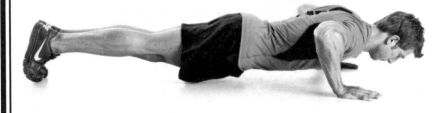

EXERCISE 2 *Pushup*

Do a standard pushup, keeping your back, butt, and legs in a straight line. If this is too difficult, place your hands on an elevated surface such as a bench or step.

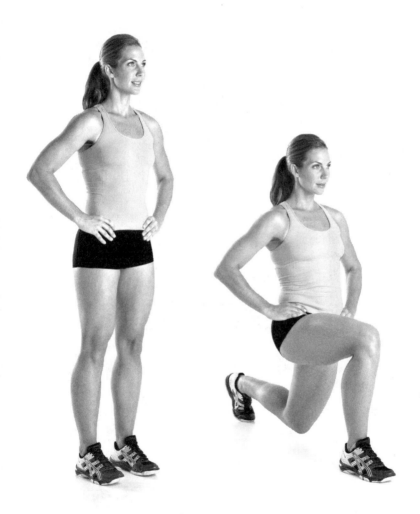

EXERCISE 3 *Right-Leg Reverse Lunge*

Stand tall, step back with your left leg, and lower your body until your right leg
(this is your working leg) is bent at least 90 degrees. Push back up.

EXERCISE ANYWHERE, ANYTIME!

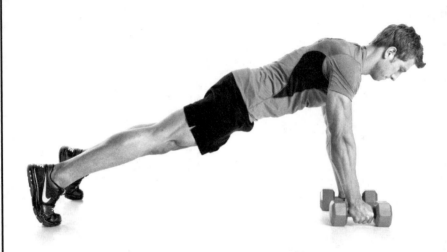

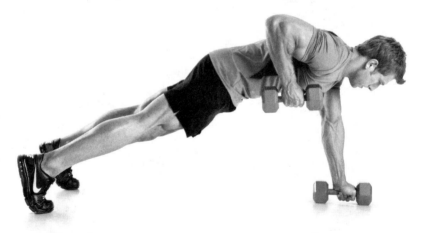

EXERCISE 4 *Pushup-Position Row*

In a pushup position (arms straight), grasp a pair of hex dumbbells. Lift the weight in your right hand to the side of your chest. Lower and repeat on your left. Try to keep your torso from rotating as you row. No dumbbells? Perform the exercise without them to build balance and strength.

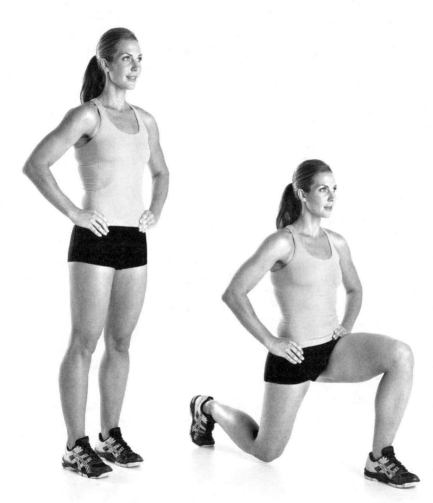

EXERCISE 5 *Left-Leg Reverse Lunge*

Stand tall, step back with your right leg, and lower your body until your left leg (this is your working leg) is bent at least 90 degrees. Push back up.

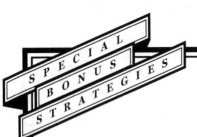

BIG EXERCISE LESSONS
WE CAN LEARN FROM LITTLE KIDS

A LITTLE MORE PLAYTIME MAY BE ALL THAT STANDS BETWEEN
YOU AND THE LEAN, HAPPY LIFE YOU WANT.
HERE'S HOW A CHILDLIKE ATTITUDE CAN HELP YOU LOSE WEIGHT.

➤ **MAKE EXERCISE A REWARD,** not a punishment. If the only time you exercise is the Monday after a dissolute weekend, then you will associate exercise with painful payback. Remember, exercise is something you should do for fun. Your dog wags his tail before a walk; build that sense of anticipation into activities you pursue.

➤ **MAKE "HAPPILY EVER AFTER" A REALITY** for those who stick to a workout regimen. That's because exercise activates brain reward pathways that act like antidepressants.

➤ **FIND MORE FUN ON THE PLAYGROUND, BE MORE POPULAR.** It's a fact: One study looked at kids who played outdoors and kids who spent most of their time indoors. The ones who went outside to play were more popular with their peers.

➤ **CAP OFF RECESS WITH CHOCOLATE MILK.** A study out of Indiana University concluded that chocolate milk is an effective and healthy postexercise drink that speeds recovery. Cyclists who received chocolate milk following an interval workout were then able to cycle 54 percent longer during their next bout when compared to men who relied on a carb-replacement drink.

➤ **EAT THREE SQUARES, TWO SNACKS.** Nutrition = energy, something no preschool pup lacks. And more energy = more workouts.

➤ **REMEMBER HOW LITTLE YOU KNOW.** You should be picking up exercise knowledge all the time from the people you see working out. If you're smart, you'll utilize what they bring. Invite it. Asking questions is how you figure things out.

➼ BELIEVE IN A BETTER YOU. You hated it when a grown-up told you, "We'll see." It's still unacceptable. Don't say it to yourself about exercise. Self-doubt will only keep you on track for an early death. But knowing that you can do anything and be anything you desire—a staple of hopeful youth—will push you toward positive change.

➼ THE WORD FITNESS DOESN'T EXIST. In the secret language of children, it's called "having fun."

➼ HOWEVER, PLAYING IS WORK. Approach your downtime with all the seriousness of a 5-year-old with a secret treasure map.

➼ FIND YOUR MOTLEY CREW. And then run wild together. You'll cover 12.5 percent more distance when training in a group than when alone, ac-

cording to research in the *British Journal of Sports Medicine.*

➼ BAN TEASING AND CRUEL NICKNAMES. Stop calling yourself Fat Ass. Be proud of what you're accomplishing, no matter the size of it.

➼ PAY ATTENTION TO HOW YOU MOVE. Early childhood is the time for checking out the working parts of the human machine. And if you pay attention to your form when running or walking, you'll improve those fundamentals of movement and help ward off injury.

➼ KEEP A PLAY AREA AT HOME. Children are 38 percent less likely to loaf when exercise tools are available at home, report Australian researchers. The same goes for you, kiddo. Make room for a few free weights and an exercise mat, at the least.

➼ TAKE BABY STEPS. Intimidated by your local gym? Feel it out

a bit before fully diving in. Stick to walking on a treadmill at first or pick out one weight-lifting machine to perform per visit. Transitions are always tough, no matter your age.

➼ STAY ON A SCHEDULE. Kids don't have a choice, and when it comes to your workouts, you shouldn't, either.

➼ REMEMBER THAT TV IS THE ENEMY OF ACTIVITY. Kids are twice as likely not to get enough exercise if the tube roots them in place for more than 2 hours a day. Limit your exposure to this dangerous box, as well.

➼ REMEMBER THAT WHAT YOU DO TODAY CAN CHANGE YOUR FUTURE. Teach a 10-year-old to play tennis, and he may still be doing it at 30 and beyond. Learn how to play golf at age 50, and you may still be walking the course at 75.

THE FAT-INFERNO WORKOUT PLAN

THIS 4-WEEK PLAN FROM ALWYN COSGROVE, C.S.C.S.,
CO-OWNER OF RESULTS FITNESS IN SANTA CLARITA, CALIFORNIA,
CAN TURN YOUR BODY INTO A FAT-BURNING MACHINE

If you've mastered the workouts in Chapter 7—even the expert version—here's a plan you can swap in that will keep your fat burn humming along. This program uses the latest training techniques to torch belly fat. You'll get an intense cardio workout, but instead of running, you'll do total-body exercises at a fast pace. After all, whether you're running or lifting, your muscles require energy to help you move. And this program of three workouts forces more of your muscles into action than you'd ever use while jogging. Not convinced? Just try it for 1 week.

Perform each workout once a week, resting at least 1 day between sessions. So you might do Workout A on Monday, Workout B on Wednesday, and Workout C on Friday.

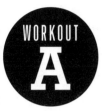

Complete these two exercises in Workout A back-to-back using a technique known as countdowns. Do 15 reps of dumbbell swings, followed by 15 reps of squat thrusts (page 214). Without resting, do 14 reps of swings and then 14 reps of squat thrusts. Continue this pattern until you finish with 1 rep of each exercise.

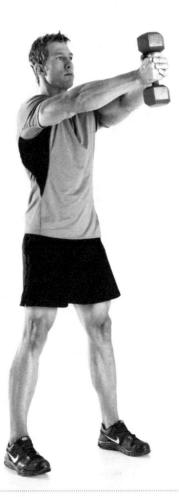

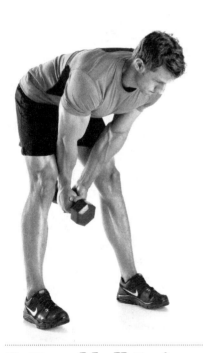

❶ *Dumbbell Swing*

Hold a dumbbell with both hands at arm's length in front of your waist. Bend at your hips and swing the dumbbell back between your legs (don't round your lower back). Then reverse directions by thrusting your hips forward and swinging the weight to shoulder height.

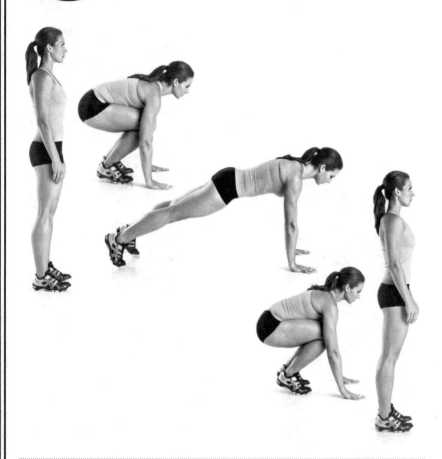

❷ *Squat Thrust*

Stand with your feet shoulder-width apart. Bending at your hips and knees, lower your body until you can place your hands on the floor, shifting your weight onto them (as shown). Then kick your legs backward into a pushup position. Immediately reverse the movement back to the squat, then quickly stand up. That's 1 rep.

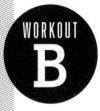

B

Perform these four exercises as a circuit, doing one after another in succession. Do 10 repetitions of each movement, and rest for no longer than 20 seconds between each exercise. Complete the entire four-exercise circuit a total of 10 times.

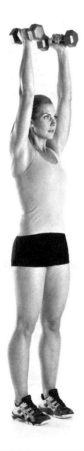

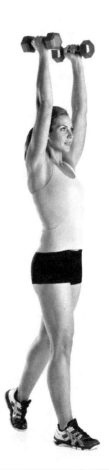

❶ *Overhead Farmer's Walk*

Grab a pair of dumbbells and press them over your head, your palms facing each other. Stand as tall as you can and then simply walk forward—each step is 1 rep. Keep your head up and stick your chest out as you walk.

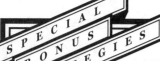
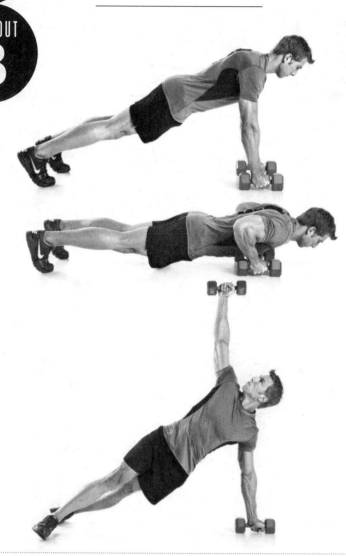

❷ *T Pushup*

Do a pushup with your hands on a pair of hex dumbbells. As you push up, raise your right arm and rotate your body toward the ceiling. At the top of the move, your arms should form a "T" with your body. Lower the weight back into pushup position, then repeat, only rotate your body to the left this time. Continue to alternate back and forth. Each pushup counts as 1 rep.

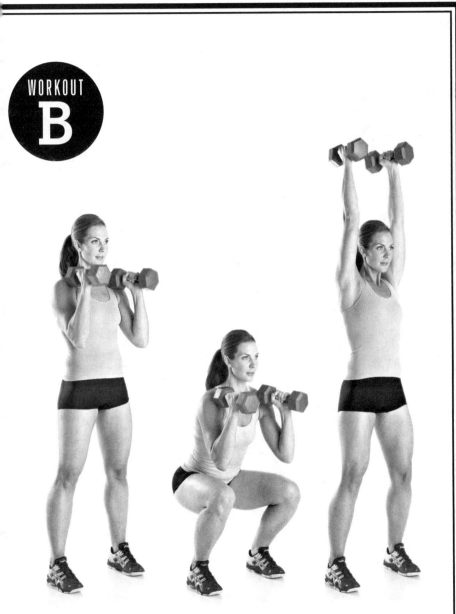

❸ *Thrusters*

Hold a pair of dumbbells next to your shoulders and set your feet slightly wider than shoulder-width. Push your hips back, bend your knees, and lower your body as far as you can. Then push your body back up as you press the dumbbells directly over your shoulders. That's 1 rep.

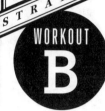
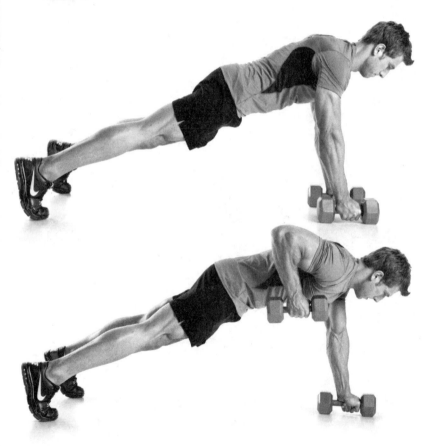

❹ *Pushup-Position Row*

Place a pair of hex dumbbells on the floor and set yourself in pushup position with your hands on the dumbbells. Without allowing your upper body to rotate, pull the right dumbbell up to the side of your chest. Pause, lower the dumbbell, and repeat the movement with your left arm. That's 1 rep.

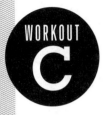

Perform these four exercises as a circuit. Do 6 reps of each movement, and cycle through all four exercises as many times as possible in 20 minutes. Rest as needed.

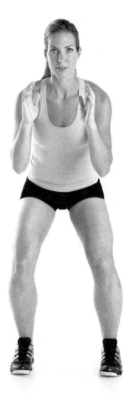
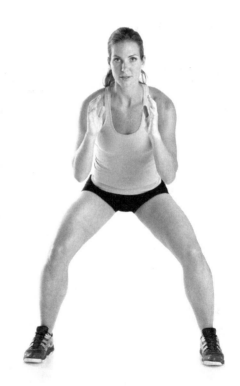

❶ *Lateral Shuffle*

Stand in an athletic stance, as shown. Shuffle 3 steps to your left, then 6 steps to your right, and 3 steps back to your left. That's 1 rep.

WORKOUT **C**

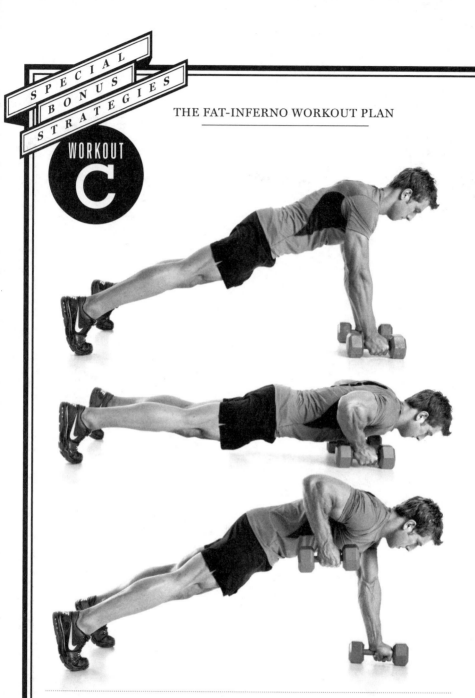

❷ *Pushup and Row*

Place a pair of hex dumbbells on the floor and assume pushup position. Perform a pushup, but once you return to the starting position, row the dumbbell in your right hand to the side of your chest. Lower the dumbbell and repeat with your left arm. That's 1 rep.

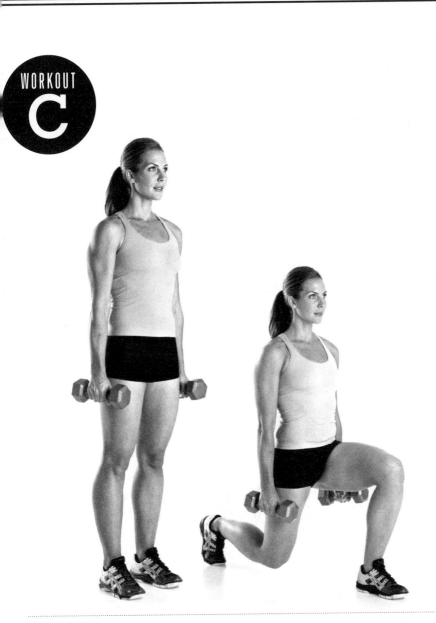

❸ *Dumbbell Reverse Lunge*

Grab a pair of dumbbells and hold them next to your sides, your palms facing each other. Step backward with your right leg and lower your body until your front knee is bent at least 90 degrees. Return to the starting position, and step back with your left leg. That's 1 rep.

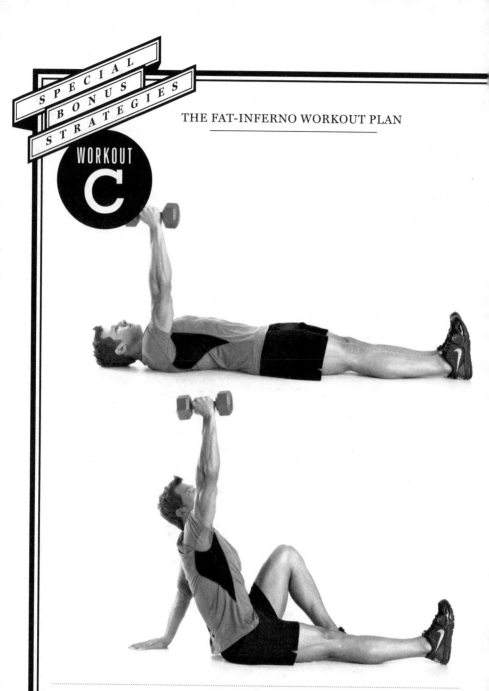

❹ *Dumbbell Getup*

Lie faceup and hold a dumbbell in your right hand with your arm straight above you. The object: Simply stand up while keeping your arm straight and the dumbbell above you at all times. Once standing, reverse the movement. That's 1 rep.

Do all 6 reps, and then switch arms and do another 6.

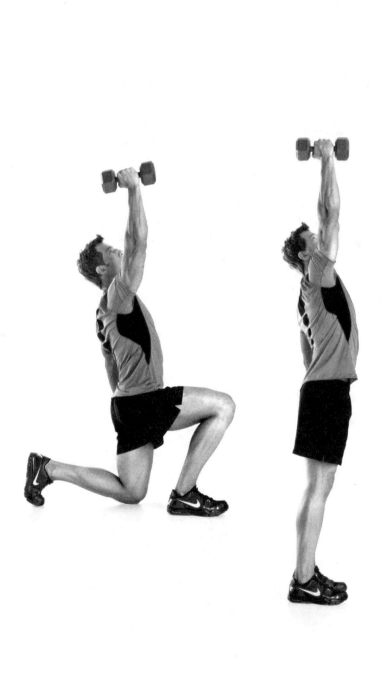

A Perfect Day of Weight Loss

You can always use your time better. Boost metabolism, burn calories, and torch your belly for 24 hours with these tips.

AM

7:00 Wake up and do 2 minutes of jumping jacks, high-knee skips, pushups, or crunches.

7:15 Have two scrambled eggs and a slice of Canadian bacon. A 2009 Purdue University study found that a high-protein breakfast makes people feel fuller throughout the day, so they're less likely to overeat.

7:45 Hit the gym, and lower weights slowly. Taking 3 seconds to lower weights during full-body resistance training can rev your metabolism for up to 3 days, according to a Wayne State University study. (Study participants used a challenging weight for 5 sets of 6 repetitions for each exercise.)

9:00 Drink some milk. A diet with plenty of calcium-rich dairy can enhance weight loss, according to a 2007 study of overweight people.

10:00 Grab a protein-rich snack, like half a turkey sandwich on whole-grain bread with Swiss cheese. In a Georgia State University study, athletes who ate three 250-calorie snacks a day were more likely to lose body fat and have more energy than those who didn't.

11:00 Walk briskly around the office/ neighborhood/mall during your break. A recent Mayo Clinic study found that lean people walk an average of 3½ miles more per day than obese people do.

PM

1:00 For lunch, eat a spinach salad with grilled halibut and sliced almonds. All contain magnesium, a metabolism-friendly mineral.

2:00 If your work meeting is with just one or two people, walk the halls as you talk.

4:00 Down a glass of iced green tea. According to a study in the *Journal of Nutrition*, the catechins in green tea decrease body fat.

5:00 Have a handful of wasabi peas or some other fiery snack. According to a 2006 study review, spicy foods help burn fat and calories.

7:00 Take a short walk before dinner.

7:30 Eat dinner. If you ate lightly today, don't worry about having a heavier meal now: "It doesn't matter when you fuel up; it's how many gallons you put in the tank," says Gary Foster, Ph.D., director of Temple University's Center for Obesity Research and Education.

9:30 Grab a good book or magazine, turn on some tunes, and relax. Stress jacks up your level of cortisol, a chemical that boosts abdominal fat.

10:30 Draw your shades so the sun won't rouse you early. According to a 2008 review, losing sleep affects the hormones that turn your appetite on and off, making you feel hungrier.

FEEL GREAT

ROLL AWAY ACHES AND PAINS

A $17 PIECE OF EXERCISE EQUIPMENT CAN
GIVE YOU AN EFFECTIVE MASSAGE
AND IT WON'T STAND THERE WAITING FOR A TIP

A simple foam roller could be your cheap ticket away from pain—
a solution just as effective as the expensive hands of a trained
masseuse. Self-massage with a foam roller ($17, performbetter.com;
the 3-foot size works well for most purposes) is all the rage—and not
just because it feels so good. In fact, it can help you exercise better
and more comfortably. That's because the roller helps stiff muscles
relax, breaks down scar tissue, and improves your range of motion.
Remember: Flexibility and mobility become increasingly important
to good health in your thirties and forties, when your joints begin to
lose some range of motion and lubrication. What's more, research
from Japan shows that people whose bodies are more limber have
about 5 percent less arterial stiffness—a marker for heart disease.

Every workout you do should start with 10 minutes of targeted self-
massage using a foam roller—it'll alleviate painful knots that constrict
blood flow and hinder elasticity in your muscle tissue. Place the roller
under your body and roll for 30 seconds over each aching muscle.
Work at whatever pace feels comfortable. It's that easy.

For a more targeted and preventive plan, try these eight moves to
ease common problem areas.

The thoracic spine,

which is responsible for your upper-back mobility.

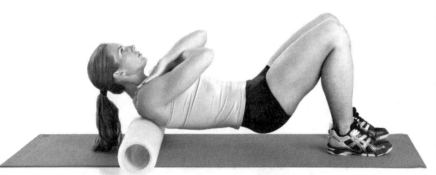

[A]

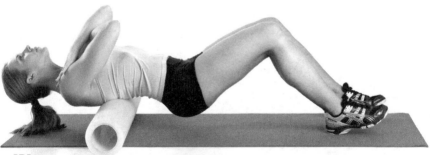

[B]

ROLL THIS WAY: Lie faceup with a foam roller underneath your upper back, at the tops of your shoulder blades. Cross your arms over your chest. Your knees should be bent, with your feet flat on the floor. Raise your hips until they're slightly elevated off the floor [A]. Roll back and forth over your shoulder blades and your mid and upper back [B].

TARGET 2

The core muscles.
They're at the root of all movement.

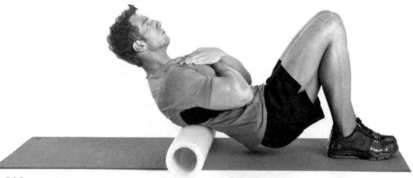

[A]

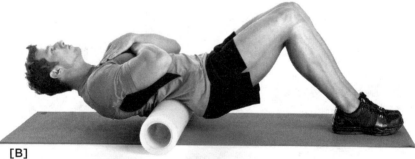

[B]

ROLL THIS WAY: Lie faceup with a foam roller under your mid back. Cross your arms over your chest. Your knees should be bent, with your feet flat on the floor. Raise your hips off the floor slightly [A]. Roll back and forth over your lower back [B].

The hamstrings,

which are major players in lower-back pain.

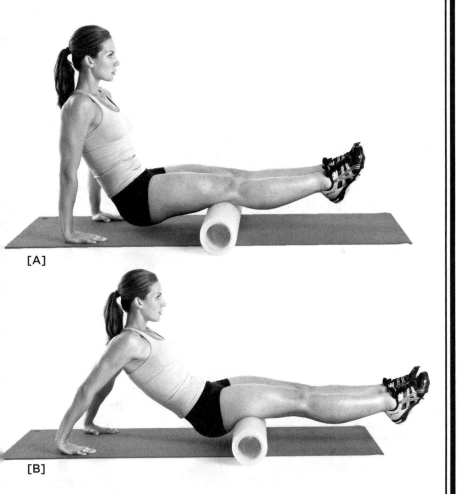

[A]

[B]

ROLL THIS WAY: Place a foam roller under your knees, with your legs straight. Put your hands flat on the floor for support. Keep your back naturally arched [A]. Roll your body forward, until the roller reaches your glutes (butt). Then roll back and forth [B].

TARGET 4

The iliotibial band (ITB),

which runs along the outside of your leg from hip to knee.
It often becomes overly tight from high-mileage hoofing
(when it's called "runner's knee").

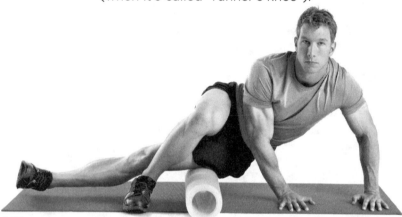

[A]

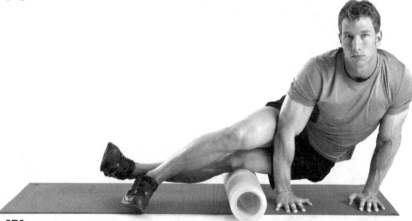

[B]

ROLL THIS WAY: Lie on your left side and place your left hip on a foam roller. Put your hands on the floor for support. Cross your right leg over your left, and place your right foot flat on the floor [A]. Roll your body forward, until the roller reaches your knee [B]. Then roll back and forth. Lie on your right side and repeat with the roller under your right hip.

The quadriceps and hip flexors.

When they're tight, they can tug on your patellar tendons, causing pain around your kneecaps.

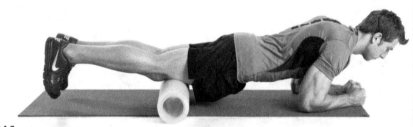

[A]

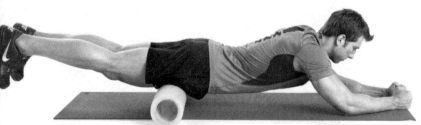

[B]

ROLL THIS WAY: Lie facedown on the floor with a foam roller positioned above your knees. Place your elbows on the floor for support [A]. Roll your body backward, until the roller reaches the top of your thighs [B]. Then roll back and forth.

TARGET 6

Your calves,

the source of the spring in your step, and your leap
on the basketball court.

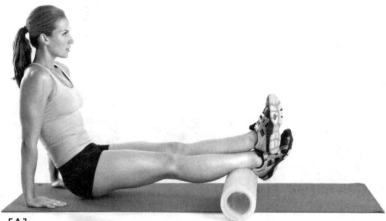

[A]

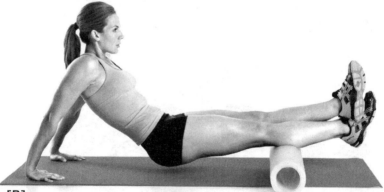

[B]

ROLL THIS WAY: Place a foam roller under your right ankle, with your left leg straight. Cross your left leg over your right ankle. Put your hands flat on the floor for support. Keep your back naturally arched [A]. Roll your body forward, until the roller reaches the back of your knee [B]. Then roll back and forth. Repeat with the roller under your left calf.

Your glutes.

Your buttock muscles are a major source of power,
plus they enhance your rear view.

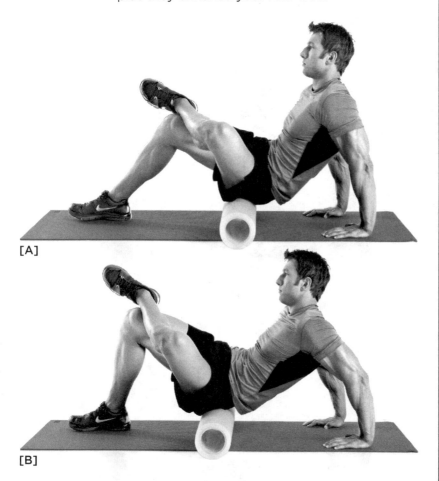

[A]

[B]

ROLL THIS WAY: Position a foam roller under your left thigh, just below your bottom, and sit. Cross your left leg over the front of your right thigh. Put your hands flat on the floor for support [A]. Roll your body forward, until the roller reaches your lower back [B]. Then roll back and forth. Repeat with the roller under your right glute (cross your right leg over your left thigh).

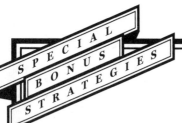

TARGET 8

The plantar fascia,

a membrane along the sole of your foot. When inflamed,
it's called plantar fasciitis. You don't want to go there.

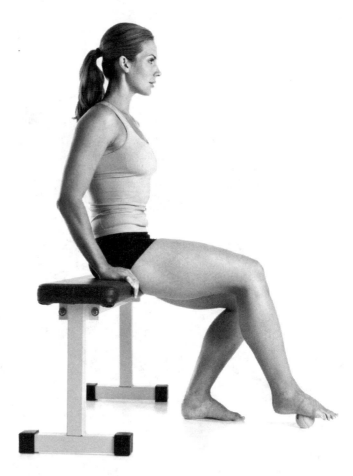

ROLL THIS WAY: Roll the bottom of your bare foot over a tennis ball. Work your entire sole over the ball for 30 seconds, and repeat with your other foot. Apply enough pressure to feel it, but not so much that it causes pain.

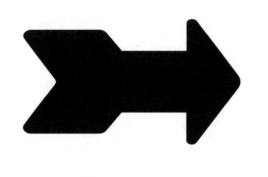

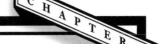

CHAPTER 8

Countdown
to a
Lean Belly

True tales of people who've won the war on fat, and how you can be the next to declare victory over belly blubber!

~~~~~~~~~~~~~~~~~~~~~~~~~~~~~~~

H ow did they do it? That's the first question anyone asks when they see a friend or colleague who's lost a lot of weight, or remade their body into a healthier, leaner version. How *did* they do it?

Well, it's no mystery. In fact, one of the most important and intriguing studies ever conducted was put together by the Centers for Disease Control and Prevention (CDC) back in 2006. This is our tax dollars at work, and I'd say we got our money's worth.

The pages of the study—its catchy title is "Dietary and Physical Activity Behaviors Among Adults Successful at Weight Loss Maintenance"—take all the world's weight-loss theories and compare them to what works for real people in the real world. It looked at people who won the fat war by losing at least 30 pounds and then *keeping the weight off* using strategies that will work for you, too.

Keep in mind: It wasn't a 100 percent success story. The CDC studied 2,124 people, and only 587 of them actually lost the weight and kept it off. But those who succeeded used many of the same strategies, the strategies outlined here.

How did they banish the fat for good? Let's find out.

WHEN IT COMES TO FOOD:

80% of successful weight losers— wait for it—ate less!

This is, of course, the "duh!" diet. I can hear the skeptics laughing right now, in fact. I'll shut them up by observing that this strategy is not as easy as it sounds, as anyone who has attempted to lose weight by reducing calories has discovered. So how is it possible that people are able to successfully eat less food? Because they employ simple strategies that circumvent hunger and straight-arm their cravings.

CHAPTER
— *8* —
LAWS OF
LEANNESS

People will try to sabotage your weight loss. Know how to answer them, and you can fight back.

The majority of successful "losers" keep the weight off by eating more fruits and vegetables.

And since reducing food intake was a weight-loss success strategy employed by a vast majority of the winners, it's critical that you, too, discover some easy ways to put a damper on hunger. Here are some creative ways you can take the technique from "duh!" to genius in a few easy steps.

Make it work for you:

PAY ATTENTION TO WHAT YOU EAT. Mindless eating is excessive eating. Researchers at the University of Massachusetts discovered that people who watched TV while they ate consumed nearly 300 more calories than those who dined without an eye on the tube. You need to pay attention to the messages your stomach is sending to your brain; if the TV is blaring, you won't see the "slow" and "stop" signs.

SLOW DOWN. Fast eaters become fat people. If you consciously stop to take a breath between bites, you can cut your food (and calorie) intake by 10 percent, according to researchers at the University of Rhode Island. Special bonus: You can do this in social situations— Thanksgiving dinner at Aunt Marge's—and nobody will even notice. That is, until you show up next year minus 20 pounds of flab.

I SAID SLOW DOWN! It takes 20 minutes for the news that you've had enough to eat to travel from your gut to your brain. The reason: Hormones that trigger the "I'm full—stop!" sensation are at the end of your digestive tract, and it takes a while for digested food to reach there. If your mouth is filled with conversation, it won't be so full of food. Talk more between bites, and weigh less when the conversation/meal is over.

BEWARE THE "HEALTHY" MENU. If you order the stuff that's supposed to be good for you, you're likely to underestimate a meal's calorie total by more than a third, according to a study in the *Journal of Consumer Research*. The restaurants know that; now you do, too. So be

Swapping good fats for bad is a weight-loss technique proven by successful dieters.	More than half of people who lost weight did so by cutting out sweetened beverages.	By far, the most proven effective "exercise" for weight loss is simply walking more.	Fewer than one in five people who lost weight needed formal exercise to do so.

especially aware when ordering "healthy", and make sure you have a "to go" box handy to carry leftovers home.

BEWARE THE COMMUNITY CHEST. Always serve snacks in a bowl or dish, and put away the packages. Never eat from the bag or container. That way, you won't ever eat an entire bag of something in a single sitting.

BEAT HUNGER WITH YOUR MIND. Have a craving even though you ate just an hour ago? Before you indulge your mystery hunger, here's how to test whether your appetite is real or not. Imagine sitting down to a large, sizzling steak. If you're truly hungry, the steak will sound good, and you should eat. If the steak isn't appetizing, it means your body isn't actually hungry. You might be bored, or thirsty, or just tempted by something you don't need. Try a change of scenery: Researchers at Flanders University in Australia found that visual distractions can help curb cravings.

71% of successful weight losers . . . ate more servings of fruits and vegetables.

This one isn't a shocker, either. So why aren't you doing it already? Use these strategies to brighten and sweeten your daily menu.

Make it work for you:

REDECORATE, REPACK, REMEMBER. If you don't have a countertop fruit bowl, buy one so you can grab a peach, banana, pear, or other piece of fruit on your way out the door in the morning, to munch on during your commute. (Plus, it's fun to throw the core out the window.) Plan a 10 a.m. apple-a-day break. Toss an orange in your briefcase to help you past the mid-afternoon lull (otherwise known as Temptation Time). Make fruit part of your entourage, and it will beat up lesser foods.

IF YOU CAN'T BEAR TO EAT VEGETABLES, DRINK THEM INSTEAD. That's right, you could have had a V8, as long as it was the low-sodium variety. It has pureed tomatoes, beets, carrots, celery, spinach, lettuce, parsley, and watercress, and 8 ounces supplies two of your five recommended daily servings of vegetables. It also heats up nicely as a base for soups.

IF YOU CAN'T BEAR TO EAT VEGETABLES, HIDE THEM IN YOUR PASTA SAUCE. And no, neither you nor the kids will notice. Using a fine grater on your food processor, grate 2 cups total of onions, garlic, carrots, beets, and zucchini (or any combo thereof), then sauté the microscopic vegetable bits in a tablespoon of olive oil. Add 4 cups of basic marinara sauce and simmer to an anonymous tomato flavor.

IF YOU'RE NOT YET DRINKING SMOOTHIES, WHY NOT? Have you read the label of your fruit juice? Lots of sugar (however "natural" it is) and not much fiber, which means it's a carb bomb when it hits your bloodstream. Not so with a blended smoothie, because ingredient number one is whole fruit, making the sugar content drop and the fiber climb. Two tips: Use frozen fruit; buy it by the bag in your store's freezer section. And buy a wand mixer and a small pitcher so you can mix your smoothie in the same container you drink it from; it's much easier than washing out a blender.

Almost any fruit-and-berry combo will do, but you can start with this recipe: ½ cup frozen blueberries, ½ banana (peeled ones freeze well), 2 tablespoons peanut butter, 2 tablespoons whey powder (it's in the supplements aisle in the grocery store), 1 cup 2% milk, and 1 cup water.

65% of successful losers . . . ate smaller portions.

The "duh!" diet, part two? In fact, maybe not, because you're probably unaware of a key inflationary trend that's been growing right alongside the national potbelly: the sizes of our dishware and glasses.

Make it work for you:

BUY SMALLER DISHES. According to the food scientists at Cornell University, people tend to eat as much food as will fit on their plates. That's where "duh!" overlaps with dangerous. Over the past 100 years, our plates have grown, decade by decade. And we also know that the nation's obesity rates have grown exponentially in that time as well. No, it's not a coincidence. If you dine off of smaller plates, you'll grow smaller, too. Shoot for 9 inches in diameter, and you'll be on your way.

DRINK OUT OF SKINNY GLASSES. As have gone dinner plates, so have gone drinking glasses. And if you fill the newly cavernous ones with any kind of sweetened beverage, you'll overindulge in calories. But here's a smart tip: We tend to gauge our drink sizes by how tall, not how

HOW TO LOSE WITH BOOZE

A FEW SWAPS CAN HELP YOU MOVE FROM BEER BELLY TO SIX-PACK

No matter how tropical your mixed drink or how light your beer, your choice of happy-hour hooch may not be as healthy as you think it is. Alcohol is still filled with empty carbs and calories that add up if you're watching your weight. Yes, what you've read about some health benefits to booze is true. Beer and wine may help ward off coronary artery disease, hypertension, and even dementia.

All of these benefits go bust, however, if you don't practice moderation, generally accepted as no more than one beverage a day for women or two for men. Learn your limit, switch to a better bar order, and raise your glass to better health.

LIQUOR

In small amounts, ethanol, the pure form of alcohol, may raise good HDL cholesterol and encourage better blood flow. Go overboard regularly and the effects reverse, increasing your risk of cardiovascular disease. The first law of liquor: Go easy. The second: Ditch drinks with inflated calories and loaded with sugary stuff.

Schnapps

This candy-like liquor is relatively low in calories, but it's usually no more than a mixture of alcohol and artificial sweeteners.

TRY Rum

Distilled from either molasses or cane sugar, this full-bodied liquor pops up most often in daiquiris and piña coladas, which, coincidentally, are some of the biggest calorie bombs at the bar. Try a Dark and Stormy instead: Mix 1 part dark rum with 2 parts ginger beer, plus a squeeze of lime. Refreshing.

Herb and Spice Liqueurs

Don't let the herbs of a Jägermeister or a Goldschläger fool you—these tipples usually contain more than 100 calories and 11 grams of carbohydrates per ounce.

TRY Gin

This liqueur packs an herbal wallop from the juniper berries that are added to the alcohol during distillation. You probably know it as a central ingredient in martinis, but it also tastes great mixed with club soda and a lime wedge. The less you do to a good gin, the better.

Coffee Liqueur

Do you know why Kahlúa tastes so good? Yep, it's packed with sugar. That's also why it contains 91 calories per ounce. Combine it with Baileys and chocolate syrup in a Mudslide, and it's like drinking an alcoholic dessert.

TRY Brandy

Brandy is full flavored on its own, so there's no need to add mixers (and extra calories). At 70 calories per ounce, a good bottle is worth the extra dough.

BEER

Resist the urge to chug: Limit your quaffing to two bottles (one for women), and you'll reap the health rewards of beer while preventing yourself from carrying around a keg of your own.

Domestic

Just because American beers tend to be brewed up on the lighter side doesn't mean they always go easy on the calories. Aim for a beer with fewer than 140 calories. Budweiser, Pabst, and Samuel Adams Boston Lager don't make the cut.

TRY Yuengling Lager (135), Busch (133), or Rolling Rock Extra Pale (120)

Light Beer

Caution: The light beer you're drinking may have more calories and less flavor than some of its nonlight competitors. Bud Light has about as many calories as regular Keystone Premium.

TRY Miller Lite (96 calories), Michelob Ultra (95 calories), MGD 64 (64 calories)

Imports

Bass, Heineken, and Pilsener Urquell all contain 150 calories or more per bottle. With plenty of other imports on the market, look elsewhere.

TRY Amstel Light (99 calories), Beck's Premier Light (64 calories)

WINE

Wine can help you live a longer life, according to researchers. Resveratrol, a substance found in grapes, has been shown to protect the lining of arteries. Some wines have more benefits than others, but whatever bottle you choose, don't feel the need to finish it. A glass a day is all you need to do you wonders.

Pinot Noir

This wine contains the highest levels of resveratrol. One study found that pinot noir had more than five times the amount found in other wines.

Sparkling Wine

Brut Natural, Brut Sauvage, and Ultra Brut have less than 3 grams of sugar per liter. Sec varieties can contain 17 to 35 grams of sugar. Doux wines contain more than 50 grams.

Cabernet Sauvignon

Moderate consumption of 1 glass of this red wine per day may help reduce your risk of Alzheimer's disease. Talk about having wine on the brain!

Chardonnay

Buy the cheap stuff. Research has found that amines, typically found in top-shelf barrel-aged wine, are the most common culprit in wine headaches. California and French whites tend to have the highest levels of amines.

A NOTE ON MIXERS Adding the wrong mixers to your drink can inflate calories and fill your glass with unwanted artificial ingredients. As a general rule, stay away from sodas and energy drinks, which contain crazy amounts of calories, and go for no-calorie club soda instead. Avoid bottled mixers, too—they're often little more than sugary corn syrup and food coloring. Use real, 100 percent fruit juice as a swap.

stout, our drinking glasses are. So if you buy tall, skinny ones, you'll think you're drinking more even though you're drinking less.

NEVER EAT FROM THE BOX, CARTON, OR BAG. Those same clever food scientists at Cornell did an experiment in which they gave one set of moviegoers giant boxes of stale popcorn and another set smaller boxes of stale popcorn. The big-box people ate more than the small-box people. The theory: You gauge the amount that's "reasonable" to eat by the size of the container it's in. Put two cookies on a plate, put a scoop of ice cream in a bowl, or lay out a small handful of potato chips on your plate, then put the container away; you'll eat far less of the treat.

60% of successful losers . . . ate fewer bad-for-you fats.

Mind you, they didn't eliminate fats altogether. Foods with fat keep your appetite at bay, and many of them are superior nutritionally to high-carb foods. Just make sure that you're selective about the ones you eat. Oleic acid is an unsaturated fat found in olive oil, nuts, and avocados, and it works to stifle your hunger, according to a study published in the journal *Cell Metabolism*. When you digest those foods, the acid is converted into a substance that helps your brain get the message to push away from the plate.

Make it work for you:

LIMIT THE FRIED STUFF. Fun fact: Fast-food burgers and chicken from KFC and McDonald's are the most frequently requested meals on death row. It kinda makes sense. The inmates won't be around to suffer the aftermath. Fried foods are packed with calories and salt, and that crunchy, oily coating beats down any nutritional qualities that whatever is entombed inside might have. That said, eating one piece of fried chicken won't be, um, a death sentence, if it's surround-ed on the plate by generous helpings of vegetables and you follow with fruit—not more fat—for dessert. What's more, the fat in the chicken will help you absorb the fat-soluble vitamins in the veggies.

EAT THE GOOD STUFF. Make sure your diet is filled with healthy fats in the forms of fatty fish (salmon, tuna, mackerel, sardines), fatty fruits (avocados), extra-virgin olive oil, eggs (among the healthiest foods known to humankind), and healthy-fat snacks (nuts are nutritional powerhouses and keep you feeling full). I even give bacon in moderation a green light; at only 70 calories per strip, it carries big flavor and belly-filling capabilities.

WEAR YOUR MILK MOUSTACHE WITH PRIDE. Milk, yogurt, cottage cheese, and cheeses all contain slow-to-digest protein and healthy fat, so they can be excellent belly fillers. And studies have suggested that the calcium in dairy products may aid weight loss. Make them part of your diet and you'll find the cow elbowing aside lesser members of the food kingdom.

57% of successful losers . . . eliminated sweetened beverages.

If you're going to follow only one piece of advice in this book, make it this one. I've said it before, but it's worth repeating: **Drinks with added sugar account for nearly *450 calories per day* in the average American's diet. That's more than twice as much as we were drinking 30 years ago.** If you're looking for a way to cut unnecessary daily calories to help you lose a pound a week, wean yourself from the overload of sugar-sweetened carbonated beverages. How? Dive into the box on page 64: "Kick Your Soda Habit." Start sampling, and don't come out until you've found three healthy drinks that can help you start phasing out your Coke habit. Start by replacing one at a time.

No, artificially sweetened sodas are *not* okay. Even if they have few calories or no calories, they maintain or *increase* your taste for highly sweetened foods, so you seek out the calorie payload elsewhere. Worse yet, they crowd out the healthy beverages. My prescription: Out with the bad, in with the great—in taste *and* nutrition.

40% of successful losers . . . reduced their intake of high-carbohydrate foods.

I'm surprised that this is as low on the list as it is. As I've mentioned, simple carbs enter your bloodstream as sugars and are likely to be stored as fat when you're inactive. They also set off a binge/crash cycle that can give your appetite the upper hand and have you reaching for the doughnut tray and candy bars throughout your day. To rein in your appetite, limit your simple carbs found in sugary drinks, processed foods, and refined breads (i.e., whole-wheat bread carbs good, white bread carbs bad; strawberry carbs good, strawberry-flavored candy carbs bad).

36% of successful losers . . . reduced their intake of food prepared away from home.

When you let somebody else prepare your food—especially if it's a teenager in a paper hat—you lose control over what you eat. And the fast-food companies, being what they are, encourage all of your worst eating habits by stuffing their products with crave-inducing ingredients like unhealthy fats, sugar, and salt. If you can stay out of the drive-thru, you can shrink your calorie intake every day.

13% of successful losers . . . kept a food diary.

Clearly, this weight-loss technique isn't for everybody. It's a hassle to write down every little thing you eat, day after day. But it's strikingly effective for those who do it. My advice: Try it for a week so you can get a handle on how many sodas you drink and under what circumstances, when you're most likely to veg out with a bowl of chips in front of the TV, and when your dessert cravings strike. That will help you identify your dietary danger zones and lead you to strategies that save pounds.

But it wasn't just dietary changes that helped all those folks lose all that weight. Becoming active was another enormous factor in leading the successful losers into the promised land of the lean (but not hungry): exercising for 30 or more minutes per day, and adding physical activity to daily routines. Clearly, these are *Lean Belly Prescription* kind of people. And that provides a great segue to talking about the activities that these "successful losers" used to shed fat and keep it off.

Here's why it's so important to keep both healthy eating and exercise going as your one-two punch against belly fat. A study published in the *Journal of Applied Physiology* reported that when people chose healthier foods and combined that benefit with exercise, they torched 98 percent of their weight directly from their fat stores. People who changed their diets alone were much more likely to break down muscle for fuel, and that's a big problem. Muscle is one of your prime metabolism boosters, so it will help you burn fat for up to 24 hours after a workout. So let's tackle the activity list, and give you strategies to make the most of it.

WHEN IT COMES TO ACTIVITY:

62% of successful losers . . . walked for exercise.

I consider that great news.

Is there a simpler exercise than walking? Is there a better way to incorporate talking with friends and loved ones into your fitness plan? Is there anything else that gets you out among your neighbors at a pace that lets you say hello? And is there anything that makes your dog happier than your saying the magic word *walk*?

A study from the University of Prince Edward Island in Canada (a lovely place for a walk, mind you) found that largely sedentary people who wore a pedometer for 12 weeks increased their total steps by 3,451 a day, to about 10,500. By walking more, they also lowered their resting heart rates, BMIs, and waist measurements.

Once you start paying attention to footsteps, you'll find ways to bank the extra strides. Thirty here, 300 there, 1,000 after dinner, and suddenly you're walking away from your old weight.

Why not start right now? The closer you pay attention, the more you'll walk. And the more you walk, the greater the temptation will be to mix in an even bigger calorie burner: running.

Lean Belly Restaurant Rules

REDUCE CALORIES EVEN WHEN YOU CAN'T CONTROL THE INGREDIENTS

Nothing is harder than staying lean when your health and welfare is at the hands of a series of short-order cooks and *Hell's Kitchen* wannabe's. Your tastebuds are their concern; your health isn't. But that doesn't mean that to stay slim, you have to be a culinary wallflower. Here are some secrets for eating healthfully even when a stranger is doing the cooking.

1 Kick 'em in the bread basket

A study published in *Physiology & Behavior* showed that people who ate a protein-heavy appetizer consumed an average of 16 percent fewer calories in their entrées than those who raided the bread basket. Pass on the rolls, and ask for a shrimp cocktail instead.

2 Beware of the booze

Because your body sees alcohol as a toxin, it works to burn those calories first—meaning that the calories in the food you eat alongside the booze are more likely to be stored as fat. And liquor makes you eat quicker, too. When researchers in the Netherlands gave people a pre-meal treat of booze, food, water, or nothing, those who got the booze ate an average of 192 extra calories.

3 Ignore the combo mumbo jumbo

At every fast-food restaurant, as soon as you decide on an entrée, you'll be asked some variation of this question: "Would you like to make it a combo meal?" Of course, you're tempted—who can pass up a bargain? But when you upgrade, you're just paying a little more money for a lot more calories—that's like giving the garbage man a tip to bring more trash to your house! People who take the upsell spend an average of 17 percent more money and receive an average of 55 percent more calories. You don't want them!

4 Focus on the foundations

What distinguishes a skinny pizza from an inflationary pizza? It's not the pepperoni, or the cheese. It's the crust. Three deep-dish slices from Domino's, before toppings, will cost you 1,002 calories. Downsize that to thin crust and you just eliminated 420 calories without lifting a finger—or giving up pizza!

5 Side with sides

Some of the best nutritional bargains at many restaurants are found on the side items menu. Black beans and rice, roasted vegetables, and mixed greens are among the best bets. Many times, two side orders will do half the damage as one entrée!

19% of successful losers . . . lifted weights.

I suspect that for 81 percent of you, the picture that just flashed in your mind was of a no-neck Bulgarian weight lifter straining as he hoisted a steel beam over his head in the last Olympics. I know that isn't you.

But you should still be taking advantage of the weight lifter's advantage: Muscle is the all-night convenience store of fat burning—it never shuts down. Not only do you burn a ton of calories while you're actually exercising, but there's also a big afterburn effect that kicks in. Your body has to expend energy to cool you down and repair the small tears in muscle fibers that happen when you lift. (Don't freak out. If you lift reasonable-size weights, you won't tear muscles, you'll just push the muscle fibers hard enough to make them grow.)

And now, for the final activity. Drumroll, please:

14% of successful losers used . . . unspecified activities!

No, that's not a mistake. I'm touting "none of the above" as an important result, because there's nothing magical about running or weight lifting or even walking. They're just the most common activities people choose in order to add more activity to their days. The only one that's important to you is one that a) you enjoy, b) fits into your life well enough that you can do it most days, and c) allows you to up your energy expenditure.

You can do that by adding three 15-minute walks to your day or by scheduling 2-hour bike rides on weekends. Or simply by walking more, standing more, lifting more, and sitting less.

Just look at your whole day as an opportunity to make the smart choices that will help you lose weight and feel better. Achieve that, and where might you be next month? Or next year? Some place far better than where you are today!

Is Walking Just as Healthy as Running?

IT'S ACTUALLY BETTER FOR YOU (RIGHT NOW).
HERE'S WHY.

There is no shame in taking an athletic stroll for exercise. It'll provide all of the advantages of running (strengthening your muscles, circulation, immune system, and your body's ability to break down harmful blood fats and stress hormones) without the risk to your joints. And research has shown that brisk walking can also help cut the risk of diabetes by a quarter. But will it burn fat? Without a doubt. The most effective workouts initially are those that last a long time (more than 30 minutes) at a middle level of intensity. Because a 30-minute walk is easier to keep up than a 30-minute run, beginner walkers lose even more fat than newbie joggers—who might already be out of breath and giving up after 15 minutes.

To build up your walking intensity, steadily increase the amount of time you walk—for example, from 15 minutes (the bottom limit for training to have any lasting conditioning effect) to 25 minutes. Then increase the number of your walks—from doing 25 minutes three times a week, ramp up to two 20-minute walks and two 40-minute walks per week, for instance. Finally, increase your pace. First, include faster phases of 60 to 90 seconds, followed by equal-length intervals at a slower pace. Allow the exertion during the faster periods to get so high that you can only do two steps per breath.

These intervals are key: They are scientifically proven methods for upping your calorie and fat burns. In time, you may want to start jogging, and when you try that higher gear, make sure to follow the fundamentals of proper running form, found on the next page.

To keep your blossoming cardio routine moving forward (and your body injury-free), follow this 10-week run/walk workout. It's perfect for novice runners, who often try to run too far too quickly. Keep in mind that one of the main proponents of the run/walk workout is none other than Amby Burfoot, editor at large for *Runner's World* magazine and winner of the 1968 Boston Marathon. If he believes in walking and running, you should, too. Each week, do your run/walk workouts on Monday, Wednesday, Friday, and Saturday, taking the other days off. The idea is to gradually build the number of minutes you run: For example, you start out by running for 2 minutes and then walking for 4, and doing that four more times. Complete the entire plan and you'll be able to run for 30 consecutive minutes—a huge accomplishment.

	Minutes Running	Minutes Walking	Repetitions
WEEK 1	2	4	5
WEEK 2	3	3	5
WEEK 3	5	2.5	4
WEEK 4	7	3	3
WEEK 5	8	2	3
WEEK 6	9	2	2*
WEEK 7	9	1	3
WEEK 8	13	2	2
WEEK 9	14	1	2
WEEK 10	30	0	0

*Finish by running another 8 minutes.

Running
Fundamentals

1 Keep your eyes focused on the ground 10 yards ahead of you.

2 Pull in your chin and stretch your neck up.

3 Lift your chest.

4 Lower your shoulders slightly and pull them back a little.

5 Pull in your belly and tighten it a little.

6 Cock your upper and lower arms at a fairly sharp angle.

7 Hold your hands in loose fists.

8 Move your elbows parallel with and close to your body.

9 Land lightly between heel and midfoot.

10 Plant your feet beneath your hips.

10 SECOND SLIMDOWN

Strategies

The food scientists tell us there are 200 decisions we make every day that impact our weight. These tips will help you pass the tests.

TRADE YOUR DESK CHAIR FOR A SWISS BALL

You've seen them, right? They're kind of heavy-duty beach balls used by exercisers to add a balance component to their workouts. It can work as a substitute desk chair, as well. "Use it for 15 to 20 minutes every hour," says sports-performance coach Charles Staley, C.S.C.S., author of *The Unnatural Athlete*. The ball will not only keep you in perpetual motion, but also strengthen your core muscles, alleviating another side effect of too much sitting: back pain.

DON'T EAT WITH THE TV ON

People who eat in front of the tube consume 300 more calories per meal on average than those who actually pay attention to what they're eating. This tip alone could save you a pound a week.

START WEIGHT LOSS FIRST THING

Researchers at Virginia Tech served overweight people breakfast on separate days. One day, they downed 16 ounces of water half an hour before eating. The other day, they simply ate breakfast. On water-drinking days, they consumed an average of 13 percent fewer calories. The difference is clear.

TAKE A BREAK TO WATCH FUNNY VIDEOS

According to researchers at the University of Maryland, watching 15 minutes of funny videos (great source: YouTube) can improve bloodflow to your heart by 50 percent and may reduce blood-clot formation, cholesterol deposition, and inflammation. Don't forget to laugh!

TRY THIS TRICK AT THE BUFFET

When you load your plate, leave spaces between each of the foods you select. You'll down about 20 percent fewer calories compared with a full plate.

READ LABELS

If the label of any food or drink in the grocery store lists more than one or two unfamiliar ingredients—the ones that look like they came from a chemistry set—put it back. Highly processed foods are filled with hidden sugars, excessive salt, and other health saboteurs. Eat simple foods, simply weigh less.

TAKE TIME TO CHEW

Chewing each bite of food for 3 seconds will allow you to savor the flavors of the food you eat, and send more satiety signals to your brain, so you'll stop eating before you overindulge.

THINK POSITIVELY

Worry increases cortisol levels, which tell your body to store fat. Smile, and slim down.

LOOK FORWARD TO WEIGHT LOSS

A study from the University of South Dakota showed that people who binge and crash focus on short-term temptations, rather than long-term gains. So if your goal is to lose weight and live better, schedule healthy snacks— celery, peanut butter, milk, for instance—for 10:30 a.m. and 3:30 p.m.

Where Do
You
Want to Be
4 Weeks from Now?

The investments you'll make today will pay off tomorrow, next month, and for years to come. Now's the time to seize a healthier, happier future—and make it your own!

W e all need a confidante, and mine is one of my closest friends, Lisa. She's also a business partner, advisor, and sounding board. I don't make a move without her, and most of the mistakes I've made in life have been made against her advice.

But as with any close friendship, there's always a little give-and-take; for all the advice on money, career, and relationships that she's given me, I've been able to pay her back with the advice she needed most: advice on taking care of her body.

Lisa and I first became friends more than a decade ago, and like a lot of friends, we lost touch for a little while as we were both trying to find our way in life. When we reconnected after years of not seeing each other, she had made herself a huge success, financially—but she had made herself a little miserable at the same time. The success came from her admirable skill with numbers, and the misery came as she watched some of her numbers—the ones that told the truth about her health—spin out of control. She had gained 20 pounds, her blood sugar was reaching treacherous levels, and her cholesterol was climbing, too. And there was another problem that she couldn't really count up: She wasn't feeling as well as she had when I'd first come to know her, just out of college.

She'd been paying attention to what seemed like the important stuff in life—starting a career, writing her personal success story—while losing track of herself in the process. While the things that defined her to the outside world, things like her job title and her 401(k), were fit and healthy, the things that defined her to herself—how she looked and how she felt—were on the decline.

Fortunately for Lisa, she recognized the problem, and she committed to making some changes for the better. (I suspect you've felt something like that, or you wouldn't have gotten all the way through this book! I applaud you for coming to that realization and for taking a step to do something about it. Nothing takes more courage than taking an honest look at yourself, not liking everything you see, and committing to change.)

$CONCLUSION$

LAWS OF
LEANNESS

Small positive gains have a way of snowballing into major, lifelong improvements.

If you do what you can, you'll soon find you can do even more.

When I first knew Lisa, back in the old days, she thought of me as her health-nut friend Travis. But when we reconnected, she'd had a change of heart. She started thinking of me as a guy who had figured out some things that were working in his life. And she realized that, heck, maybe some of them would work in hers, too.

She looked around for a couple of things she could do immediately: a healthy food here, an opportunity for exercise there. She noticed how these changes made her feel—better! more hopeful!—and thought, Why not make a few more changes?

As a businessperson, she was well aware of the idea of compound interest: how if you save the equivalent of a few bucks a day (I didn't like waiting in line for that latte anyway) and invest it, you're soon earning money on not only the original stake, but also on the profits that stake is throwing off. The small gains soon take on a life of their own, and later on in life, you can live off the investment.

I'm telling you this story because the idea of changing your life is sometimes overwhelming. Fortunately for Lisa, she had already seen how you can build financial health by making small steps, day after day. Now she was ready to do the same thing for her body.

I put together an easy program for her—the same kind of program I've put together for you. No crash diets, no crazy exercise programs, just small changes each and every day. And for Lisa, those few small commitments paid off in small ways—Hey, those jeans fit me again!—so she made more. And as she made more changes, and bigger ones, she felt capable of doing things she hadn't thought would be possible. The after-dinner walks became runs, the single food swap became a whole new way of eating. It wasn't a shock to her life, it was more like a gradual transformation propelled by how much better she felt as the process went along.

Focus on what you can do today, and tomorrow will take care of itself.	Studies show that after just 4 weeks, healthy lifestyle changes become habits.	Fitness investments are like financial ones— they yield returns for years to come.	You're just one simple move from starting the best part of your life: the future!

That's what I wish for you, as well. I won't blame you if you feel a little overwhelmed by the sheer number of strategies I've proposed to you over the course of this book. I did that not because I expect you to take on all of them, but, rather, because I know nobody can. I don't even do all this stuff. What I do is what I can, and what feels right to me, and what feels sustainable.

That's where I want you to start. Decide on your PICK 3 TO LEAN choices from Chapter 4. Stick with them for 4 weeks. A cool study I read tells me that you can form a new, healthy habit in that amount of time.

Do the same with the activity levels I prescribe in Chapter 6. Schedule that walk after dinner most nights, and plan an adventure every Saturday morning for the next 4 weeks. I'm not asking you to sign up for the New York City Marathon. At least not yet. I want you to do things that won't hurt you, that you'll feel good about, and that you can do with your immediate circle of friends and family. No pressure on you or them, just a gentle question: Is your current state so great that it couldn't use a few new alternatives that make you feel better?

Lisa felt the prodding toward progress, and she'll never turn back because she likes the way she feels and looks now. She brought out the better self she knew existed inside, and moment by moment, decision by decision, improvement by improvement, she shook off the old self who was headed in the wrong direction. I'm talking about incremental change—bit by bit, not leap by bound.

Many of us experience incremental change in the negative direction. We don't remember the moment when we became shrouded in a fat layer because it slowly built up over the years as the metabolism fire dimmed and our reliance on processed and fast foods increased. There was no shocking moment while looking in the mirror, because the weight gain happened slowly. By the time your doctor starts talking to you about your weight or the health problems it's causing, you may feel like it's too hard to turn a tide you didn't notice in the first place.

It's not.

Put your faith in the stories of others who've succeeded—many of them with weight problems worse than yours. They'll tell you that you can't drop 30 pounds in a month or two, and I'll tell you that it wouldn't be healthy to try. The people who lose weight and keep it off do it by committing to the gradual life changes they can live with long-term and that will pay off in the months and years ahead, not minutes.

They see it as finally being good to themselves in a meaningful way, rather than taking sugary rewards that may please for the moment, but doom them to painful years later on in life.

I want you to focus on what you can do today. Right now. Build your success story one small triumph at a time. One useless food exchanged for something that really satisfies. One new activity that transforms time you'd spend vacantly staring at a screen. One connecting point between you and your family that sets you all in motion and builds your relationships at the same time.

I'm talking about making your life richer and more fulfilling while you're casting off bad habits you probably don't feel good about anyway. And you're not going to do these things because I tell you to, you're going to do them because they make you feel and look better. And remember, those two are one and the same.

You're one simple move away from starting the best part of your life, which lies ahead. Just one small change that makes all the rest possible.

INDEX

Underscored page references indicate sidebars and tables.
Boldface references indicate photographs.

E

F

N

O

P